Anna's Story

and:

New Effective Treatments For Rheumatoid Arthritis

by

Richard L. Lyonharte

First Edition

1999

ISBN 978-0-7414-0204-2

INFINITY PUBLISHING
1094 New DeHaven Street, Suite 100
West Conshohocken, PA 19428-2713
Toll-free (877) BUY BOOK
Local Phone (610) 941-9999
Fax (610) 941-9959
Info@buybooksontheweb.com
www.buybooksontheweb.com

Dedication

This book is dedicated to all those who suffer from the agony of severe Rheumatoid Arthritis and to the doctors, spouses, and friends who hope and pray for the victims of this affliction. It is hoped that this will help in some small way for all.

Preface

My credentials for a medical text are meager, to say the least. Nevertheless, with the help of many medical texts, books, the Internet, and my training as a researcher, I feel I managed to gain some insight into the nature of the disease and provide some real help for sufferers. There was something driving me to do this ;why is hard to explain. I worked all day at work ; rested for about an hour; and worked at home until about 1 or 2 A.M. To this day, the source of this energy is unknown. Something in me or beside me provided the inspiration and the drive. I feel certain that there are much better medical texts , but this one has feeling. Whatever you do, you will not regret the time spent reading this ,even if, at times, the reading is not so easy. Two of your fellow human's very beings and Souls are opened to you and their struggle for life. It is not a trivial tale. The book is written in the hope that it will help those who suffer from Rheumatoid Arthritis, especially the very severe form.

Table of Contents

Anna speaks to us from a place where all is good. She desire to help us and hopes that she will be remembered . This information is to help and is critical and important. Let Anna speak !

Hello, my name is Anna and this is my story. All that you read is true. I am now with God. My husband is writing and speaking for me. This is a story for you and may make you think. Please think of all the people that suffer and help them. You may cry; you may smile; you may wonder; you may discover yourself; but you will not regret reading this. This will be an experience that you will never forget. Please read on……

"She was a Phantom of delight
When first she gleamed upon my sight;
A lovely Apparition, sent
....
A perfect woman, nobly planned,
To warn, to comfort, and command ;
And yet, a Spirit still, and bright
With something of an Angelic Light. "

She Was A Phantom of Delight

by

William Wordsworth (1770-1850) (some text omitted)

This and other poetry begins to express the nature and being of Anna. She was a joy to be with and a Treasure unlike any ever before or after on this earth. At least this is the way I felt.

Introduction

This is a book about a courageous woman and her affliction of Rheumatoid Arthritis (**RA**) . The disease was particularly severe in its effects and progression. The effects of the medicines used for treatment almost equaled the effects of the disease. Severe **RA** is now called by some as SADS or Severe Arthritic Disease Syndrome ; most just refer to the disorder as **RA** which may be a mistake since the effects and the progression of the disease are much much pronounced. In many countries such as Finland and many others, tests have been developed to identify such a form of **RA** and use the most aggressive treatments early in the initial stages to limit the harmful and eventually fatal results of this form of **RA**. Anna had ,in addition to **RA**, Crohn's disease which must may have occurred after the **RA** by about 8-10 years ,but which appears to have a strong link.

The progress in research on this autoimmune disease in the last two years has been both prodigious and phenomenal. Using the Internet as well as conventional texts, many new developments have been identified. These developments include many older but not widely used treatments as well as very new medicines. In addition to the new medicines are new treatment protocols that should be of help. The work identified should help all with **RA**, and someday this disease as well as many others will only be found in textbooks.

Chapter 1

The Storm (Disease) and Its Effects Develop

We usually wait for a storm. It is so much better then. I'll start with one of our favorites. It is best if read with the correct feeling.

Annabel Lee by Edgar Allan Poe (This has been changed slightly from the original)

"**It** was many a time ago,
In a kingdom by the sea,
That a fair maiden there lived-whom you may know
By the name of **ANNABEL LEE**;
And this maiden she lived with no other thought
Than to Love and to be loved by me."

This poem was followed by others by Poe especially *The Bells* and of course, *The Raven*. This was accompanied by Wine and Cheese and all manner of Activity that befit the night and mood. Our love equaled that eloquently described by Poe and the experience was to cherish all the events, and our love, which still shines with a Light both there and on earth.

" But thy eternal summer shall not fade
Nor lose possession of that fair thou owest:,
Nor shall Death brag thou wanderest in his shade
When in eternal lines to time thou growest;
So long as men can breathe, or eyes can see,
So long lives this, and this gives life to thee."

William Shakespeare

Just before God took me into his Eternal Love, my husband and my Love spoke with the Angel of Death. It was a short conversation ,but he certainly remembers it.

“ *Richard* “ spoke The Angel of Death, *“She has suffered enough.”*

God’s Angel informed him in a Commanding but Fatherly Manner that it was time for me to leave.

The following is a letter I sent to one of her many doctors. Their efforts, the nurses, and the hospitals were prodigious in their efforts to save her and make her life bearable. The disease unfortunately had no real cure or effective treatment.

Richard L. Lyonharte
111 Main Street
Metro City USA

Dr. Specialist,

Thanks so much for kind and thoughtful note. We all miss Anna (Lou). She was such a joy in my life and a constant source of happiness and contentment. She really liked you and the treatment you provided. You are a superb surgeon and Doctor. I was very impressed by your work ; if there had been some effective treatment for the Rheumatoid Arthritis, the outcome would have been quite different. I really miss Lou and always will. I also appreciate the tender care given to her by you and the many doctors she had. Being a Doctor is a noble and caring endeavor ; the rewards of helping others would be immense. I wrote this just after Anna’s Funeral Service :

Anna (Lou) was the light of my life and brightened the very presence of all the people she contacted . Lou was good and made you feel good. She is with God now ,and I am sure she and the rest of the Angels are having a great time. Her Love and the strong feelings we had for one another will live forever. I still love and cherish her and the kindness and Love she exuded. She made all people feel a little bit better. That will last, and someday we will be together again. I feel most fortunate that she did marry me ; the last 22 years were a constant Joy to me. I am very lucky; I know what heaven will be like since I have experienced it for the last 22 years. I know that you may have experienced some of this and know that this will last. She lives in my heart and thoughts and with God forever.

My sincere and everlasting thanks for your caring and care.

Richard L. Lyonharte

Chapter 2

The Many Forms of Autoimmune Disease

There are many diseases and disorders of the human body ; **R**heumatoid **A**rthritis (**RA**) is just one of many of the autoimmune diseases. There are many immune disorders and you may be surprised to learn that there are so many. Some are listed:

1. Rheumatoid Arthritis **(RA) :**

    1. **Primary to this discussion and identified by bold type**
    2. Juvenile RA
    3. Psoratic Arthritis
    4. Ankylosing spondylitis
    5. Lupus
    6. Sjogrren's Syndrome
    7. Goodpasture's Syndrome
    8. Reiter's Syndrome
    9. Progressive systemic sclerosis
    10. Vasculitis

The following are specific to a certain organ, but are still autoimmune disorders

Heart

1. Rheumatic fever
2. Dressler's Syndrome
3. Postmyocardial infraction syndrome
4. Postpericardiotomy syndrome

Endocrine System

1. Addison's disease
2. Hasimoto's thyroiditis

3. Diabetes melitis

4. Graves disease

Blood or Hematological

1. Autoimmune neutropenia
2. Thromocytopenic purpura
3. Pernicious anemia
4. Autoimmune hemolytic anemia

Neurologic disorders

1. Multiple sclerosis
2. Myasthenia gravis

Gastro-Intestinal disorders

1. Chronic hepatitis
2. Inflammatory bowel disease : Ulcerative colitis and **Chron's Disease (CD)**
3. Primary billary cirrhosis

The list goes on and on. If immune deficiency is added, the list gets bigger; "Have you ever heard of AIDS ". If allergies and skin disorders are added, the list gets even bigger. One sad effect of these disorders is that the door is opened for other disorders and diseases that may much more serious or fatal.

Would it surprise you if many of the treatments for **cancer** were used and indicated for immune disorders? The reasons why will be explained later. It should be obvious that this category of diseases is large and well known to both doctor and patient on a very large scale. If **RA** is discussed, it must be discussed in the context of the family of disorders that encompass the disorder. Many of the texts and many of the so called " Miracle Cure" books only discuss the specific disease and the wondrous discovery of how to cure the malady. There is a link between disorders in a common category. The link is expanded when it is realized that many treatments for other disorders also work for that disorder.

Chapter 3

The Influence of Microbes on Human Life

We live in a sea of apparent and not so apparent organisms. The animals and plants that we easily see are categorized as to good or bad and behavior and their use to us. The good guys are easy to distinguish from the bad guys. In the same vein of thought, we pay much attention to members of our species and make similar judgments . There are good, bad people, and definite threats. Even collections of people give similar considerations to the other groups of the same species and classify their behavior and actions. This behavior may even take the form of war and involve the mass killing or destruction of many humans.

The real enemies (and friends) cannot be seen by the unaided eye and may only be observed with optical or electron beam microscopes. These organisms may exist at our peril such as some bacteria and many viruses . Some of the organisms exist in harmony with us and are essential to our life. All of us ,if we survive, are equipped with a system that will defend us, around the clock tirelessly, and destroy the foreign invaders. The immune system is our greatest defender against a large host of micro organisms. The immune system kills or disables the foreign invaders; some of our own cells that are useless or damaged are disposed of; and the useful cells that comprise **Self** are recognized and retained. This is the function of the normal immune system. The immune system is structurally comprised of the Thymus , the Spleen, The Intestinal associated lymphoid tissue, Special Tissue in the Bone Marrow , and the Lymphatic System with the Multitude of Lymph Glands, and the lymphatic fluid in the blood. The lessor (and sometimes enlarged or diseased) components are the tonsils and adenoids. These are usually but not always removed.

“**G**ather Ye rosebuds while you may,
Old time is aflying;
And that same flower that blooms to-day ,
To-morrow shall be dying .”

Lord Byron

RA usually develops unknown to the patient. Some symptoms may be present early, but usually not. There may be some fatigue; there may not. There may be a persistent low grade fever, but again there may not. There will definitely be vague, but noticeable pain and some swelling in the joints in particular the feet especially the bottom or heel or ankle. There may be some pain in the back or in the hands or elbow. If the **RA** is severe, noticeable swelling will be present and may be very painful at times. If the **RA** is mild these symptoms may also range from vague to noticeable to slightly painful. The symptoms may and will expand to the hands, particularly the fingers. The wrist, elbows, knees, and ankles may become profoundly painful and stiffen with use. The symptoms are very noticeable in the morning and after some activity of the previous day. There may some edema in the feet and ankles but only when some activity has preceded. Later, the symptoms will appear even at rest with no apparent cause. The joints will also feel hot. You may also have increased fatigue and sometimes a slight weight loss. ***See a physician immediately!***

Tests for RA

The doctor will make some tests. These are:

(1) An Erythrocyte (red blood cell) sedimentation rate test. This will show as an elevated level.

(2) A complete blood count will reveal moderate anemia ; the white cell count may be high or low not "normal"; and many others which reveal abnormal functionality.

(3) X-rays will show some bone demineralization (after some time); the soft tissue swelling may not require X-rays

(4) Analysis of the synovial fluid from the joints shows a very high white blood cell count as well as a turbid appearance.

Your doctor at this point may refer you to a specialist such as a Rheumatologist . Your own doctor may decide to treat you ,but he or she will probably order additional tests. The specialist will also require additional tests. The doctors will also do a detailed physical examination. The tests are for increased levels of Rheumatoid Factor (RF) levels (this will be explained shortly) and there will also be an elevated serum globulin level. The doctors and test personnel are quite good at this part of the disease analysis and treatment.

You will be informed of their findings. Much testing must be done to determine exactly which immune disorder you have. Once the diagnosis is clear, the patient is informed.

It is not the end of your life and much can be done at this point. It is critical that you keep your hopes high for there is much that can be done for you at this point.

Chapter 4
Treatment of RA

There are many drugs that will give real relief and are very effective. This information is repeated briefly and may be found in almost any book on RA. The old standby, aspirin works quite well , and will give some relief. There are many others that are called Non Steroidal Anti-Inflammatory Drugs (NSAID) and include such drugs as: ibuprofen, acetaminophen, , and others. There are other NSAIDs that can only be obtained by prescription. There is a very good reason many of the following can only be obtained from your doctor with a prescription-They all have moderate to severe side effects.

1. Ibuprofen- May also be prescribed by doctor, product name is Motrin by Upjohn
2. Indomethacin , product name is Indocin by Merck Sharp & Dohme
3. Naprosyn , product name is Naprosyn by Syntex
4. Tolemetin sodium with a trade name of Tolectin
5. Sulindac , trade name of Clinoril by Merck Sharp and Dohme
6. Prioxiciam ,trade name Feldene by Pfizer
7. Melclofenamate sodium with a trade name of Meclomen
8. Diffunisal, trade name of Dolobid by Merck Sharp & Dohme

And the list goes on and on.....

BEWARE THAT THE MORE EFFECTIVE THE NSAID THE MORE SEVERE ARE THE SIDE EFFECTS. This is not a trivial warning. Some of the very effective drugs can do severe damage to you.

The side effects may be minor such as headache, or they may range from acute **g**astro**i**ntestinal (GI) damage such as ulcers and bleeding to possible acute renal failure. Follow the directions to the letter and take with food and milk as directed. If buffered aspirin works use it ; use whatever works with a **minimum** of side effects. Be fully aware that ulcers and other GI damage is very possible and may range from barely noticeable to severe.

Before proceeding to outline the rest of the medicines for RA. A very brief description of the disorder will be given. Later a more detailed description of the disease will follow.

***Anna's story continues*…….**

We met in 1976; I and my **ANABEL LEE**. My life was literally transformed by her being. Ours was truly a love that was more than love. Our life was pure pleasure in unimaginable ways. Our happiness knew no bounds and surely even the **A**ngels smiled.

" **I**f all the world and love were young,
And truth in every shepherd's tongue,
These pretty pleasures might me move
To live with thee and be thy love.
Time drives the flocks from field to fold,
When rivers rage and rocks grow cold,
And Philomel becometh dumb;
The rest complains of cares to come.
The flowers do fade, and wanton fields
To wayward winter reckoning yields;
A honey tongue, a heart of gall,
Is fancy's spring, but sorrow's fall.
Thy gowns, thy shoes, thy beds of roses,
Thy cap, thy kirtle, and thy posies
The coral clasps and amber studs,
Soon break, soon wither, soon forgotten,--
In folly ripe, in reason rotten.
Thy belt of straw and ivy buds,
All these in me no means can move
To come to thee and be thy love.
But could youth last and love still breed,
Had joys no date nor age no need,
Then these delights my mind might move
To live with thee and be thy love. "

The Nymph's Reply , Sir Walter Raleigh (ca. 1552-1618)

We were married in the Kingdom by the Sea (Actually the city is very well known, and is by the sea) . My being and life was truly transformed. Our love was such that life was transformed into a magical state that no one could possibly imagine was possible. This state of bliss lasted until 1981. After returning from a trip, Anna experienced very painful swelling of her feet, general overall pain, and pain in her hands and wrists. The severe swelling disappeared after about three days. We went to see a doctor and he conducted a series of tests including Sedimentation rate, X-rays, and others as previously described. He informed us that Anna most likely had Rheumatoid Arthritis (**RA**) and referred her to a Rheumatologist. The Rheumatologist conducted additional tests and verified the initial diagnosis.

" **A**nd it was the reason that long ago,
In this kingdom by the sea,
A wind blew out of a cloud, chilling
My beautiful **ANNABELL LEE;**"

Annabel Lee Edgar Allan Poe (1809-1849)

Chapter 5

RA Defined

What is this **RA** ? What malady can produce such prolonged and unremitting suffering and transform being from pleasure to pain ? What disease is this ? Why does this occur ? Why me ? Why my wife-my love ? Why ? These questions seemed valid to me, but only some of the questions have answers.

Remember we live in a sea of foreign organisms that are not all benign. To survive, we have immune systems that fight, kill, and destroy these organisms. The immune system is our internal army-even some of the cells are called NK (natural killer cells). The buggies (viruses and bacteria) are shown no mercy and promptly dispatched and carried way for disposal. Hooray for our side !

Unfortunately, the immune system sometimes makes mistakes. Serious mistakes-mistakes that are not rectified. For some reason, the ability to distinguish Self is lost, and the immune system attacks the good guys-US ! Our internal army can do much damage and it does and it **NEVER** stops or rests. We have no reserve army and no secondary system to stop the immune army gone berserk . In a way we are under attack by nature's most perfect and well trained and disciplined army. There is no escape-we hurt, we swell, we are gradually being destroyed.

This explanation is not found in most texts and a more conventional explanation follows. Most texts explain that the cause of **RA** and many other auto-immune disorders is not known. But there are some theories and some models. In the past two years, even the past three months, some amazing research has been revealed. This will be explained and well as current treatment for RA. A Tower of Hope and possible Salvation is being erected by a great army of dedicated and talented doctors, researchers, and scientists. As Sherlock Holmes was fond of saying, " The game is afoot Watson !" Indeed it is ! We shall sometimes be masters of our destiny. This is a sacred promise in some of the most revered works of man and God , and we enjoy the great privilege of living in this era of enlightenment.

RA is characterized by the formation of altered very specific immunoglobulin antibodies known as altered IgG that are formed when the immune system is exposed to an antigen. An antigen is any substance that can induce an immune response. Usually this caused by the bad buggies. In the case of **RA**, it is our own cells that cause the effect- Bad Scene Man ! The body's immune system forms a defensive response (antibody) against, **itself in mass**. This antibody, which should not be formed, but does for some unknown reason, is known as the RF factor. The RF factor forms in mass aggregates to such an extent that massive internal damage starts to occur. This destruction and joint damage, in particular, attracts some serious leukocytes (white cells) that can greatly magnify the damage and cause severe pain and inflammation. The battle is on ,and your own army is hell bent to destroy not just the bad guys (the buggies-bacteria, viruses, etc.) but **YOU !** This is indeed a serious situation that must not be taken lightly. One of the most efficient and ,on a comparative basis, one of the largest armies is attacking, and the sole objective of this army is the destruction of **YOU ! Thus, the doctors and you must fight with whatever is available.** The internal situation can be modified and mediated .

Thus, as harmful as the current medicines are, they must be used until more effective measures are available. The good news is that these new treatments are close to being perfected .

Chapter 6

Current and Available Medications

For : Daily Living and Coping

There are many medications and treatments available from your doctor or Rheumatologist. The **NSAIDS** have been presented in some brevity . There are many other medicines and classes of medications that **may** mediate or control the disease. Actually these medications may appear to control the symptoms of the disease but the internal army is still at work ; you may have just slowed its work.

There are categories of **RA** that may be apparent or may not be apparent at first. The moderate or mild form of the disease or disorder is amenable to treatment. The severe form is also responsive to treatment at first. Sometimes the mild will change into severe ; it is rare for the severe to ever change.

Daily Routines

If you have RA or are caring for someone that has RA or simply helping someone with severe RA, there is a lot that needs to be done. There are many good books on this and some of the best are from the major universities and/or medical schools or the Arthritis Foundation. Read what they publish and apply it religiously. This information is merely a supplement that has been learned by caring for someone with severe **RA**.

Firstly: They (or you) hurt and all the time. Getting out of bed is major chore. All of the simple tasks of daily life are painful. The proper medication as prescribed by the doctor or doctors must be taken early in the day and thereafter as directed by the physician. Eat a low calorie and healthful diet. You will want to have an intake of at least 1000 mg of calcium and a plentiful supply of potassium. The lowly banana is a good source (your doctor may prescribe potassium chloride). Cremes and ointments that promote circulation help. A warm shower or bath will help. Rest if tired. Hopefully you can get out of bed. If you can, moderate exercise will help. Walk around the block-do something. You may want to rest again. If the **RA** is not too bad ,you can usually pursue a vocation that you enjoy. If not consider hobbies that keep your mind and body active. The main idea is too keep yourself active and your heart healthy. The only way to do this is to move. Move your arms, move your arms, move yourself-but Move. It will hurt but the payoff is to keep your heart and circulation healthy. If you have a spouse, let him or her give you a gentle massage. This will greatly help your lymph system circulation. As the day progresses, your metabolism will increase and you will usually feel better.

If at possible, use a good warm indoor pool, and do aquatic exercises. This will do your body good with a minimum of damage since the water supports most of your body. You will require rest ,and if you need it ,a short nap does wonders. Your activities must make you happy ,and promote your well-being and social contacts. You may love certain very specific activities. These may be painful but your health will benefit. The books and phamplets published by the Arthritis Foundation are very good at providing very helpful information.

The medications you take will help the **RA**, but they do suppress your Immune System and they do affect your skin and vascular system (especially the Corticosteroids). You must, later in the disease progression, provide protection for your lower legs and lower arms from impact damage. Simple impacts will do a lot of damage and care must be taken (Consult Appendix B) . Thin leather protective devices may be made or purchased for your lower legs and arms. You may use Velcro fasteners and make the protective coverings decorative and compliment your wardrobe . For emergencies, consider the use of thin ACE bandages. A puncture wound to a person with **RA** on an array of Immune- suppressive medications is a serious event . Consult your doctor immediately. The wound may appear to heal and actually be the source of a major infection. Show it to the doctor ,and usually a strong antibiotic will have to be used if there is an infection. Always take even minor wounds seriously.

Of all the weapons against **RA**, the most effective is your own mind and spirit. Do whatever makes you happy. Simple daily activities help. Do not give up. Progress is being made daily and this disease will be conquered.

Corticosteroids

Corticosteroids are clones of natural hormones produced by the adrenal glands. Their use goes back almost 50 years. The drugs are used to block or slow steps in the allergic and inflammatory response caused by the defective immune system . Your berserk army of white blood cells produce some compounds that can be mediated or suppressed to some extent. The medicines will make you feel better but there is a price to pay. The **Corticosteroids** depress the immune system and over a long period of use produce some side effects that may not be desired to effects that can be just as dangerous as the immune disorder itself.

There are also glucocorticoids, and adrenocortical steroids. The drugs include prednisone, prednisolone, metylprednisolone, hydrocortisone, and dexamethasone. They are very effective for other conditions such as transplants to suppress rejection, for psoriasis, certain eczema's, and even certain cancers. In addition, the drugs are used for other immune disorders such as Multiple Sclerosis, Lupus, and many others. In addition, the medications are used for Chron's disease and ulcerative colitis. This list may just touch on the use of these medications.

If used with care and in mild doses, these medications do help with inflammation and pain. The joints also appear to function better-at least the pain is mediated. There are some very serious problems with long term use; if suddenly withdrawn, the patient may collapse with severe pain, etc., perhaps proceed into a coma, sometimes die (rare). The problem is that the body's production of these hormones is suppressed; thus the patient must continue the medication. Thus, as stated earlier, there is a price to pay that may not be acceptable. For this reason and the long term damage effects, most current treatment practice is to limit the intake on a long term basis to about 10 mg a day. Unfortunately, this may not be adequate for patients with severe **RA**.

For a low dose (or a high dose) the most noticeable and first effects of the medication are increased appetite and weight gain. Next there will be an increased retention of salt and water. Next ,the patient becomes more sensitive to infection and damage by simple impact. The skin thins and weakens; simple bumps into furniture and other impacts turn into major problems with infection being a common complication.

There are other problems but quite so serious as the previous. These include increased or elevated blood pressure (not always); muscle cramps (may be controlled); insomnia; extremely thin skin that is easily damaged or bruised; cataracts ;and osteoporosis. Surgeons have very strong opinions and refer to prednisone and the like with a preface of **Damm !**

If you don't like what has been offered as help , there are more medications. These can be very effective at first, and if you have mild **RA**, they will work (at least they give real relief). The drugs most used first are usually those with the mildest side effects. If you are one of the lucky ones, this is all that will be needed (at least, at first).

Plaquinil

These medications are called disease modifying since it was thought years ago that they indeed did modify the disorder. The first to be tried is usually (but not always)hydroxychlorine or (Plaquinil-Winthrop-Breon). This is used to treat Malaria and is very effective for Malaria. This drug takes a long time to work if it does work at all. Mild side effects include skin rashes, loss of hair, headache, blurring of vision, ringing in the ears, nausea, stomach cramps, and diarrhea. More serious side effects include loss of vision, excessive muscle weakness, anemia, decreased white blood cell count, and infection. Usually, unless the RA is mild, the Plaquinil is totally ineffective, and a waste of time (which is a very valuable commodity for the patient).

Sulfasalazine

Another mild agent is sulfasalazine that is also used for ulcerative colitis. This may help if the RA is mild; usually this is also a dead end medication with no relief especially if the **RA** is severe.

The usual course of therapy is to try these medications first since the side effects are tolerable , at least for a short time. In many other countries, there is a classification process. If you are determined to be in the mild category, then these medications are tried. However, if your **RA** is severe, ***all of these are not tried (or should not be) since time is a very vital consideration and an effective treatment must be obtained as quickly as possible since the damage is so great every day.*** The unseen army is hard at work and attempting to eliminate offending parts of **Self**. Thus, for the patient with severe RA, this investigative approach is very damaging and should be bypassed since time and minimizing damage are important.

If you are the patient you have every right to ask if you have mild or severe **RA**. If the answer is not forthcoming-**Find another doctor**. **Your time is valuable, and day to day pain and inflammation is not acceptable.** Einstein and Newton frequently referred to the fabric of time and life as woven with this fabric. You only have limited time, if healthy. If sick with **RA**, time is very limited . Effective treatment **must** start as quickly as possible. If the treatment is effective, your time allotment increases. Unfortunately, many doctors do not go to what is most effective at first since the medications that work have very ,very serious side effects. Thus, the current thinking is to be cautious; but some texts refute this and advocate much different approaches.

"Dost thou love life ? **Then waste not time**, for **time is the stuff that life** is made of."

Benjamin Franklin

Peniclliamine

Another interesting medication is peniclliamine (**Depen** by Wallace**)**. Copper, mercury, and lead poisoning such as Wilson's disease (excess copper) are treated with this drug. This is also sometimes effective against **RA**. The use of this is not widely favored but it works on all forms of **RA**, but after a short time (from 6 months to about a year) ceases to be effective. The side effects are possible kidney damage, blood and bone marrow toxicity, and muscular weakness. There is some evidence from John Hopkins University that this medicine will work if a certain genetic marker is present. However, the usefulness of this is limited for a short time and X-rays may show that damage is progressing and something else must be tried. ***Is the tune familiar ?***

The tune is played over and over and runs like this:

***Well, this is thus and that is that and where we are is at :* " We need to try something else. Your case is most unusual. But we have many more drugs we can try ."**

***Well, this is thus and that is that, and where we are is at:* Let's try it again, and again**

(Play with gusto and repeat again and again and again) ……………………

God in Heaven ! The X-rays and tests show the patient being destroyed. The **A**rmy of the **B**erserk **I**mmune (**ABI**) marches on and on . Havoc and pain reign supreme inside the patient's body, and the doctors play as if this were a unique case ,and over and over the **" Platitude Song" is repeated.**

Well, this is thus and that is that, and where we are is at:

Let's try it again, and again (***Play with gusto and repeat again and again and again)***

Well, this is thus and that is that and where we are is at : **" We need to try something else. Your case is most unusual. But we have many more drugs we can try ."**

Well, this is thus and that is that, and where we are is at:

If you hear this too often **<u>seek another doctor</u>**. You do not have infinite time and your **Self** is being destroyed by the **ABI.**

Gold and Gold Salts

These medications are next used, and are the old but heavy guns of the Rheumatologist. These medicines will have a definite effect. As a matter of fact, Gold (salts) do aid about 50% of the patients as long as they can tolerate the side effects ,and these are very severe for a large portion of the patient population. The gold is given first by injection. One common reaction is the skin comes off in your mouth ; another is a severe rash ; another is a rash and itching; More serious side effects are serious kidney damage and bone-marrow suppression. If you don't have these effects, then some great relief is possible.

Ridura

If the injections cause too serious a reaction, the gold salts can be given orally as Ridura-Smith Kline & French. This is much safer than the injections and a much lower incidence of side effects. Blood and urine tests must be conducted to evaluate possible damage. Most can tolerate this medication.

A combination of NSAIDs, a low dosage of cortisone, and one of the DM drugs may appear to be the answer to the disorder ,and appear to give some tolerable life. Unfortunately, the **Army of the Berserk Immune** (**ABI**) is still at work and continuous monitoring of this unwanted activity is necessary as well as tests for the adverse effects of the medications.

You may still experience pain ,and increasingly, less use of your joints. It is now time for the Nuclear weapons of the fight against the **ABI**. These drugs are really powerful and can help. They can also kill you by inducing a cancer, destroying your liver, and other effects that may make the preceding medications appear as candy.

Cytotoxic Drugs

These drugs were developed and are used to halt or control cancer cell growth. Hence the name Cytotoxic ; the drugs alter or stop cell division ,and the T cells and helper cells die. This is a potentially dangerous scenario that may cause great problems for the patient. The key words here are **use**, but with great **care** with controls and monitoring. Some are also used to prevent organ transplant rejection. Some of these can definitely cause a cancer. Some will disable your bone marrow. Some will destroy your liver. The major side effect is **death**. When the tune is no longer played or you say you still need help, the big guns are rolled out. These medications are impressive and some really work and will really help you. These drugs include the following:

1. Azathioprine-aka Imuran by Burroughs Wellcome

This drug is used to block the immune system to prevent tissue rejection. It will work in the most severe **RA** if the patient can tolerate the side effects. These include nausea that is unlike any other you may have thought possible. There are drugs that can help with this. Some of the helper drugs are very new or under investigation. This drugs works by severely depressing the white blood cells. This effect makes the drug potentially seriously toxic since your Immune System may not properly respond to an attack by bacteria or virus. The other side effect is easy bleeding and bruising which is vastly complicated by Corticosteroids. As a matter of fact, this can lead to a fatal Cancer. The old devil and deep blue sea effect.

2. **Methotrexate** (***Golden Boy***) **This medication really works and can produce dramatic improvement. If used in low dosage and with certain other treatments, this will help. Unfortunately, sometimes the liver damage is so severe that the medication must be stopped. If used early in the disease and with the proper dosage and combined with other DM drugs and NSAIDs, the improvement is dramatic.** Sometimes, the damage to the liver is such that this must be stopped in about 2 years, sometimes, the patient can take this for up to 10 or more years. **It is my opinion that his drug be used early at a low dosage and in combination with others for severe RA. Later some new drugs will be introduced that rival Methotrexate or may be used in combination with this medication.**

This drug is not a true immunosuppressive or Cytotoxic drug and deserves its own category, but is included herein since it is potentially toxic. The drug works by interfering with the way cells use and absorb, etc. nutrients such as Folic acid in particular. Thus, Golden Boy will slow down the activity of the ABI and provide real relief to the RA patient. It really works and is the focus of much work and is used by many. In addition, it acts to inhibit the activity of the ABI in the synovial membrane that lines all the joints. Thus it gives fast -fast relief, and the patient immediately responds.

It is easy to take-injections are not required. ______ <u>It works and works well.</u> The side effects are mild except for the Liver damage (fibrosis). You must discontinue drinking and smoking to use this drug, but it works- so life is better. Unfortunately, about 10% have serious side effects and must have the dosage reduced or if the liver damage is severe, the drug must be discontinued.

3. Chlorambucil a.k.a. Leukeran by Burroughs Wellcome This is used in the treatment of leukemia ,but may give pronounced relief to very severe **RA .** The danger is the severe depression of the bone marrow, and it is a known carcinogen. These side effects limit its use, but with care the drug is of use, since most of the side effects are reversible.

4. Cyclophosphamine a.k.a. Cytoxan by Bristol-Myers. This drug is effective and will help but has serious side effects. The adverse reactions are anemia, bone marrow suppression, pulmonary fibrosis, elevated liver enzyme levels, and thromocytopenia and leukopenia. These side effects especially the last two can be severe. This compound will bond directly with DNA and can cause permanent genetic damage. This and the other effects make this drug one of last resort by many doctors. It will help with vasculitis. The drug also interferes with cell growth and division-hence its use for Cancer. It is also Cytotoxic . In addition to all of this, it also kills lymphocytes.

5. Cyclosporine by Sandoz and others. This is used for the prevention of organ rejection after surgery. It is also very effective in **RA** . Some of the side effects are headache, nausea, edema, nephrotoxitic reactions, hepatoxity, and pain. Blood tests are indicated with close monitoring. This may be very useful in cases of severe **RA** when response to other medications is poor. This drug selectively works on helper T cells and B cells . This does not affect the bone marrow and is safer than many other immunosuprressives. This was to be tried next for **Anna.**

There are many other drugs in all categories . Some are better, and some are worse ,and some do little at all. Consult booklets from the Arthritis Foundation for the latest medications. Most all have side effects that range from mild to severe to even worse. Thus, a qualified physician is an absolute necessity .

Anna's Story Continues ......

Anna was on almost all of the above medications except for the last two, Leukeran and Cytoxan. Her treatment was extensive, and by more than one physician. She was in the hospital a number of times, and was considered to be in the very severe **RA** category. At first some of the medications helped. The only NSAID that really helped was Feldene. Later there was an high price to be extracted on the body for this help. Prednisone was used at up to 25 mg per day. There was a very high price to be extracted on the body for this help. Peniclliamine did help for a while . Most of the medications worked a little ,but after trials were ineffective.

Then the Great Wizard of the North saith " Ye must partake of Golden Boy (Methotrexate)" Behold great wonders. The Princess is better; the Sun again shines. Life is Good. ... But Immense Clouds start to appear. .... A great Chill occurs- Golden Boy must leave.

The use of **Methotrexate** was so beneficial ,and Anna had a semblance of a normal life for a while until a liver biopsy revealed damage to be starting that could be a real problem. Later, **Imuran** was tried as well as gold salts by injection, but the side effects of the **Imuran** were so severe that it had to be stopped. The gold salts by injection caused the skin in her mouth to come off; it, too was discontinued. The toxicity of a lot of the medications is severe. If well or if the **RA** is mild, the body's tolerance may be better and their use may be tolerated with success. Some of the very new medicines under test ,and in an experimental stage, may have helped , but were unavailable at the time.

Within the last two years, the science and techniques and medicines available, under development, and under consideration, has made the Science of Immunology almost blossom like a field of flowers just after a much needed rain. I will describe some of this, and the very real hope that is quickly moving into the realm of reality. In the short future, **RA** and many of the auto- immune disorders will become history . Life will be better. The medications and treatments and discoveries are developing so rapidly that quickly available resources that can be accessed (by booklets, by the Internet, and by Research Foundations) are listed for current inspection.(see Appendix A) . These people are doing work that is exciting and very meaningful. This is a new frontier that is being explored , and conquered with a quiet enthusiasm that easily equals the effort in the 60's to go to the Moon. The benefit to us all and future generations will be immense.

Chapter 7
Disease Severity Increases

Anna's Story Continues ....

Anna had very severe **RA.** In addition, we found later that she had some concurrent problems with GI problems. The magic wrought by **Golden Boy** had to be discontinued since the liver was being damaged . A series of extensive tests including a liver biopsy were conducted. The liver was starting to get spongy , and **Methotrexate** had to be discontinued. Oral Gold (Rheumatex) helped somewhat but her condition rapidly deteriorated. A slight increase in Prednisone helped. Feldene helped with the pain and inflammation but did little to arrest or even slow the progression of damage. Imuran was tried, but her nausea was so severe ,along with other symptoms, that it too had to be stopped. Injectable Gold Salts were tried again but caused all the skin in her mouth to fall out. Next, more severe Cytotoxic drugs were tried but the severity of the side effects was so great plus no improvement, that they too had to be stopped. The progress in Research present today was not in evidence at the time. Meanwhile the **ABI** was at work. The damage being done was essentially unchecked.

She found that increased bed rest did help, but no long relief was obtained. There is a very distinct difference in severe **RA** and milder forms of **RA.** The milder form of the disorder responds to a lot of the medicines; the severe **RA** only responded to the strongest medications which were also very toxic. **Methotrexate** worked. I think some of the others would help if the side effects were not so severe, or some medicine could have been given to control the side effects and toxicity. The battle was being lost ; self was destroying self. No one knew why Anna had **RA** **,**and the medicines were ineffective. Just before she died , the doctors were to start with the Transplant medicines such as Cyclosporine.

Meanwhile, we found that she had a combination of Ulcerative Colitis and Chron's disease plus severe damage caused by Feldene-ulcers, etc. An emergency Ileostomy had to be done. Anna lost about 2-3 pints of blood from the rupture of the intestine before the operation could be completed. After massive blood transfusions and removal of the part of the intestine, she started to get much better. It was a real miracle that a surgeon could be located quickly; that he was not only good but the **Best Surgeon** possible; and the apparent exchange of whole blood stopped the **RA.** After recovery from the surgery, there were no **RA** symptoms for about 2 months. Unfortunately the disorder returned.

Some new phenomena started to appear. Her skin became very thin and was easily infected. Edema started to appear in her ankles and legs. Mild at times, and very severe at other times. Her reliance on her bed became very pronounced. A low residue diet plus a low salt diet helped, but the edema and infections were persistent. Our life changed dramatically. I thought this was as bad as it could get-the worst was over and her condition was certain to improve. This was in error- the worst was yet to come.

" **O**ur revels now are ended . These our actors,
As I foretold you, were all spirits, and
Are melted into the air, thin into thin air;
And like the baseless fabric of this vision,
The cloud-capped towers, the gorgeous palaces,
The solemn temples, the great globe itself,
Yea, all of which we inherit shall dissolve,
And, like this insubstantial pageant faded,
Leave not a rack behind. **We are such stuff**
As dreams are made on, and our little life
Is rounded with a sleep.

From *The Tempest* by William Shakespeare

Chapter 8

CURRENT THERAPY

The really good therapies are still in the lab or under test. Some will be available shortly; others may require many years to be approved by the FDA ,and undergo all the required clinical trials . Fortunately, some of the laws regulating this process are being modified, and the approval process may be greatly accelerated. Some may be obtained by participating in a clinical trial organized by NIH (National Institute of Health) and many others.

For the current time , the **NSAIDs** are useful and do help with secondary symptoms and directly aid in the control of inflammation and pain. The **Corticosteroids** are useful and can help but should be used at doses that are in the 10 mg, range per day; unfortunately this may not help and the dose may have to be increased. The **Corticosteroids** can give pronounced but temporary relief if injected into the affected joints. The gold salts, **Penicillamine**, **Plaquenil,** and many others in the second line of defense category may help if the **RA** is mild. If the disease is mild, almost any of these medications will give some relief to profound relief. If none of this helps, the patient has progressed to or has had severe **RA** all along. There are currently good techniques that are used to identify the disease.

If the patient fails to respond to most of the milder therapies, the **RA** is severe. About 50% of patients fall into this category, and the severity may follow a bell curve index. Careful analysis of high contrast CT X-rays or better yet, the knowledgeable use of **MRI** can easily make the disease progress evident. There is a test that can identify the severity of the RA. A test originated in Finland by Jokien and coworkers have they devised a very high confidence method. They use Epstein-Barr virus in a culture of stimlated lymphocytes. A high Ig production will indicate with a 90% confidence that the **RA** is severe. The test is very simple and inexpensive Details may be found in *The British Journal of Rheumatology* , 33 (10): 917-22, Oct., 1994. The authors may be contacted at the University's Cell Biology Department. This test is so reliable and simple that it should be adopted as a universal standard. **It is NOT currently used in the US- WHY NOT ?** There are other tests ,and these may be adequate. If the **RA is severe the the use of DMARD or the Cytotoxic Drugs is clearly indicated. DO NOT WASTE A TIME IN PROGRESSING TO THIS STEP IF THE RA IS SEVERE. The patient is much better and able to tolerate these drugs if he or she is relatively good condition. If done quickly (under two years), the patient may become much better.**

It is recommended that the following doctors be used :

(1) A **Primary Care MD** such as a general practictioneer **.** This doctor will do the day to day care and advise the other doctors as well as be advised by the other doctors.

(2) A **Gastroentrologist**. The severe GI side effects should be monitored and tracked by this doctor.

DO NOT WAIT UNTIL A CRISIS DEVELOPS !

(3) DO an MRI or high resolution CT scan. Use a **Radiologist** if the definition and disease damage is hard to define.

(4) A **<u>GOOD Rheumatologist</u> is ESSENTIAL. This is the BIG GUN that must be used.**

(5) Consult with a **Heart Specialist**. Make all required tests.

(6) <u>Do</u> the Finnish **RA** Severity Test-Or some equally acceptable test.

The patient or their Caregiver must make these arrangements. Your MD will recommend a Rhematologist, and if you like, the other needed doctors. Make the appointments and do and take what these doctors recommend. If you are not getting better, the essential change is a new Rheumatologist. Since the **RA** may be severe, it is essential that this determination be made early.

An exercise program must be initiated. This will be very simple. First, walk some or until you feel the need to rest. Simple topical ointments can help with the pain and give some relief. The **best** exercise is water immersion and swimming, if possible. This does wonders for your whole body, especially the heart and lungs. Since, the majority of your body is supported by the water, the damage potential of this exercise is low and your heart and lungs will love you. Be moderate, but do this on a regular basis. It is **CRITICAL** that you keep your heart and lungs in shape. No matter what your heart and lungs need the best of your attentions. Curiously, these organs get better if exercised properly.

If you smoke-**STOP !** The nicotine restricts the blood flow in critical areas and does much harm. The effect on the lungs is well documented.

Wine in moderation is OK ,but avoid large intakes of 80 proof or higher drinks such as Gin, Vodka, Burbon, etc. This , in moderation, is marginally accetable unless you are on Methotrexate. This and other drugs impose a large toxic burden on liver. Do not drink at all if on these medications. It may be OK for you to have one glass of wine ,or one beer; this may be of some help but do not exceed this very moderate intake.

If find that you have trouble sleeping, and if you find that the illness is causing some depression, then an antidepressant can help. One of the side effects of some of the older medications is you will feel sleepy and rest vey well. These compounds are known as tricyclic antidepressants are have been around for some time. They will help ,especially to obtain a good sleep.The drugs in this category include Amitriptyline, Desipramine, Doxepin, and Trimipramine. Your doctor is best able to decide which is best for you.

One of the simplest ways to keep informed is to obtain phamlets from the Arthritis Foundation and subscribe to *Arthritis Today.* The magazine is free with your donation of $20 or more. Donations to the Arthritis Foundation are your best hope of assisting those that are actively seeking to help you. The address for the Foundation (local) may be found in your telephone directory. The National Office can be found at:

Arthritis Foundation Inc.
1314 Spring St., NW
Atlanta, GA 30309

The treatments mentioned before as under development may be availiable in the near future.

There are many treatments that are heavily adverised as cures that have very little value. If you have very mild **RA**, the treatment with Tetracycline may help. If you have mild **RA** , for some reason, most of the conventional therapies give good relief. If you have common osteoarthritis , many of the so called cures will help. One that is heavily advertised is glucosamine sulfate. This has been used for years to treat animals and has been found to be of some value if you have an osteoarthritis problem ; it has little or **no** effect on severe **RA.** The other treatments are herbal, fish oil, nutrition,etc. These may help, but not much. The greatest benefit is to the seller of these.

Magnetic (except for MRI) and laser treatments are to be avoided. The magnetic field has no effect (ultra strong magnetic fields excluded), and the laser beam can harm the skin severely. Copper bracelets cannot hurt, but they are useful only as jewlery. There may be herbal remdies that may help but read the literature carefully.

There are some treatments that may be in the quasi-experimental stage that may be worthy of mention. These are described by Alan S. Cohen in the text *Progress in Clinical Rheumatology* , Vol. 1. This is published by Grune and Stratton, Inc. The text may be found in most clinical libraries. Of interest are the unusual treatments for **RA** that are described in Chapter 4. Your Rhematologist will be familiar with these. The use of Cytotoxic drugs is discussed at first (1984) but then some other therapies are discussed. One of the first is "Thoracic Duct Drainage". Another is "Apheresis" which is described in detail. The next is "Total Lymphoid Irradiation " which is also of interest . These treatments never became popular due to cost and risk , and the need for very special equipment. The current texts rarely

Anna's Story Continues........

"**R**emember me when I am gone away,
Gone far away into the Silent land;
When you and I can no more hold by the hand,
Nor I half turn to go, yet turning stay.
Remember me when no more, day by day,
You tell me of your future that you planned :
Only remember me; you understand
It will be too late to counsel them or pray.
Yet if you should forget me for a while
And afterwards remember, do not grieve ;
For if the darkness and corruption leave
A vestige of the thoughts I once had,
Better by far you should forget and smile,
Than that you should remember and be sad."

From *Remember Me When I am Gone Away* by Christina Rossetti (1830-1894)

The disorder known as severe **RA** is quite different from the mild version ,or even from the associated disorders such as ostheoarthritis. The latter is one we all get, if we live long enough. **RA** ,especially the severe version, is in a class onto itself. The prognosis is not good for the long term at present.

The disease has many cousins and additional complications. One of the **greatest** dangers is to the patient's **heart**. The long term effects are very noticeable. Edema is one of the first signs that the heart is in trouble and cannot properly move the blood and lymph properly. Anna experienced this as well as many other problems. The lower legs are severely affected. Be aware that the patient is very fragile in this area and must be protected. I found that wrapping the lower legs with ACE bandages was very effective in preventing cuts and bruises when the patient was moving about. (*This is repeated again for emphasis*) . A simple cut must receive immediate attention since it can easily progress into a serious infection. This happened on more than one occasion, and I learned that protecting the integrity of the lower limbs and forearms was **critical**. A more fashionable approach is to make a simple covering from thin leather, and use Velcro to fasten the leather to another band with Velcro. Another problem with the edema is the lungs-be aware of developing problems (especially potential pulmonary edema) and **keep your doctor informed** .

The **ABI** attacks the joints; and the hands and feet will require surgery. This can be done and usually is very effective. Major replacement will be required, eventually, of the hip in particular. Anna experienced all of this. Her hands were rebuilt . Her feet ,especially the toes, were redone. The surgeons did marvelous work. The replacements and repairs were impressive. The hip replacement is a major procedure, but results in restoration of limited mobility (for Anna). This was one of Anna's major surgeries. Unfortunately, the drain on the body is severe ,and she got much worse after the hip surgery. Limited mobility returned but the **RA** got dramatically worse. **Imuran** was tried again but was of little help since she got so sick that it was impossible to keep up the therapy. The edema got profoundly worse (heart is beginning to fail).

Additional problems with the back which had earlier been minor became major. X-rays revealed serious deterioration of the lower spinal column. The **RA** was actively attacking the disks. Another problem was severe pain from compression of the Sacral nerve. The pain was severe and required much medication for relief.

The next problem was a secondary problem with Chron's disease. The lower intestine became completely blocked, and the Ileostomy had to be redone twice. Anna survived all of this ,and appeared to be doing better. Then one day she was having great difficulty in breathing- her heart was failing. In the hospital, with the proper medications, and about 6 liters per minute of pure oxygen, she improved dramatically. The edema and associated problems disappeared in about three days. She now had a new set of additional doctors. The heart problem was known as Congestive Heart Failure. A combination of a diuretic (**Furosemide**) and Digoxin (**Lanoxin**) with the pure oxygen was very effective. Anna got better and came home. Her use of the oxygen was eventually decreased to 3 L/min. and she appeared to be much better. Her prognosis appeared better.

Of all the diseases that receive attention as potential threats such as Cancer and many others, it is very surprising to note the lack of attention given to the potential threats caused by **RA.** It is common to hear someone refer to their osteoarthritis problems in terms of pain, etc. as a major problem. They seem to oblivious of the extremely serious nature of severe **RA.** MS and other diseases receive great attention but not **RA.** The public needs to know that this disorder is in the same league as MS and Cancer-It is not a killer per se but it can result in mortality . Even if treated, the long survival rate is not good. Only about 18% of the patient population live beyond 15 years with severe **RA.**

The trivial nature accorded the disease by the public is a real problem since the general perception is that it is a minor disease-***It is a Killer*** , and the public should be properly informed. Accord the same respect for severe **RA** that you do for Cancer (a life of only 1-6 years). The major difference is **time**-you have more time (15-20 years) with **RA** , but it is a painful and difficult time.

Chapter 9

The New Treatments-A Layman's Guide

I tell you,

Ask and it will be

Given you:

Seek and you will find;

Knock,

and it will be Opened to you.

Luke 11: 9 King James Bible (slightly modified)

This is not a medical text but much what will be presented is very technical. I will try to condense the work ,and give full reference as to who did the work, where, and possible future information. If some of this can be used, ask your doctor. You may be pleasantly surprised to hear that he or she is also very much aware of this work ,and has been following the progress for sometime. The sequence of presentation will not necessarily be in chronological order.

A Simple Observation

One of the observations I made , and that all surgeons know is that just after a major surgery where at least two or more pints of whole blood had to be administered, the patient with **RA** after and during recovering will have a much improved immune response and will for about 2 months appear much better. This has been known for some time. A possible therapy then would be to replace the whole supply of about 13 pints with blood from a healthy donor. This has been done at Duke University and other research centers. It works, but unfortunately, the **RA** reappears (usually, but not always).

BMT: Bone Marrow Transplantation- An Old Technique Refined

An old, but also a new technique, is bone marrow transplantation. This has been used to treat cancers and immunodifficiency disorders for a number of years. Recently the technique has been proposed for **RA** and is in clinical trials for Multiple Sclerosis. This work is being coordinated by Dr. Richard Burt of Northwestern University , Seattle. Dr. Burt is a leading advocate of the use of bone marrow transplantation for autoimmune diseases. This work is described in the Cellpro web site located at **http://cellpro.com.** Basically, the stem cells in the bone marrow are replaced with healthy new stem cells and a new immune system is created without the characteristics of self destruction of the old. Cellpro is actively seeking patients for the MS study and for future **RA** studies, will probably be seeking volunteers with severe **RA**. You may contact Cellpro at **312-908-800** or Fax to **312-908-0028.**

Cellpro, Inc. is located at:

22215 26th Avenue SE
Bothell, Washington 98021.

They have an **800** number of **221-2778.** They have successfully treated over 5,000 people (for cancer) with outstanding results. The process is described in many periodicals as well as on the Internet. If you need financial assistance, or if your insurance carrier has problems with funding, there are special programs being set up. It is best to contact Cellpro. The President of Cellpro, Inc., Richard D. Murdock had a fatal cancer. He was one of the first to try his therapy; **he is alive and very well.** He was recently on ***Good Morning America*** **on ABC TV** . He is an inspiring speaker . There are many programs and many new drugs-**THIS ONE WORKS !** The treatment is the final stages of approval by the FDA. The use for autoimmune diseases is just starting.

Please be aware that this is still considered in the experimental area in the United States and the treatment will require special arrangements. **The treatment is approved for many cancers but its use for autoimmune disease such as MS and RA is still in an experimental stage**. This status may rapidly change, and by the time this text is available, this treatment by bone marrow transplant and T cell -depleted autologous stem cells may be available. The treatment is a much more advanced state in Europe and Canada.

Dr. Curt Civin has been doing exceptional work in the same area at John Hopkins University in Maryland. This treatment uses stem cell grafts that will not trigger immune rejection. This bone marrow transplant technique has been used in Europe and Canada. More than 1000 people have been successfully treated. The **RA** and Lupus trials should or have begun. This work may be found on the Internet ; the keyword to your search would be John Hopkins University (JHU). This should have FDA approval soon and the work is done in conjunction with the National Institute of Health (NIH). Information may be obtained from Elise Hancock at JHU.

Thus, a previously dangerous procedure with a mortality of about 4-5% is now becoming relatively safe and extremely effective. I feel certain that others are actively pursuing this therapy and many more research and treatment centers may be working on this or have this treatment in the near future. **CellPro's** treatment is in an advanced stage of development .

Other treatments are developing that are designed for use by your physician with the method of administration being simply injection or orally. Thus, when approved, these may be done by a simple visit to your doctor. At present, the therapy may be obtained by enlisting in a clinical trial. JHU and the NIH have very large programs and are seeking volunteers. Most medical institutions and Clinical Research Institutes have clinical trials. A list in the appendix is provided of potential sites. Some medicines and therapies may be obtained by your own physician if he is willing to follow the required tests and documentation, which may be very demanding (Note, this has **recently changed**). The following touches on some of the more well publicized medications and treatments. Those medicines and treatments that are in a mostly laboratory and preliminary clinical trial are covered later .

New Drugs and Protocols

Immunex , a biopharmaceutical company, heavily involved in immune technology and science, has developed a medicine known as **Enbrel.** This drug has been under test for at least two years. This drug uses a an enzyme with a bound metal ion that performs a **t**umor necrosis factor-**a**lpha **c**onversion by the **e**nzyme. Thus, the acronym **TACE**. This has been licensed to Wyth-Ayerst research of American Home Products. The TNF is a natural immune system protein. Too much TNF leads to the cascade effect of RA. This effect as well as other will be explained later. The drug **Enbrel** can bind with the excessive TNF. This stops the cascade effect, reduces swelling, pain, and tenderness. In addition, the side effects are well tolerated. This drug must be under further trials but appears promising. Recent trials as reported by Dr. Larry Moreland of the University of Alabama are very encouraging. The inhibiting action of the biological effects of TNF seem to be possible with only minor side effects that quickly disappear. The study is actively supported by **Immunex Corporation.** Recently, Immunex reported that the drug had been used successfully for juvenile rheumatoid arthritis (**JRA**). This was reported by Dr. Daniel Lovell, MD, of the Children's Hospital Medical center of Cincinnati, at the American Academy of Pediatrics' Pediatric Rheumatology into the Next century meeting . The drug is now in Phase III trials for adults. More details may be found in the text of Dr. Lovell from the Meeting Proceedings. The success rate was 76% improvement. There have been many press releases recently about **Enbrel** ; most are from Dr. Lovell and the **Immunex Corporation.** This information may be obtained in detail from the company or on the Internet.

Another drug is out of Canada and is called **Bispan.** This was developed by Inflazyme Pharmaceutical Ltd. This company has many special formulations for inflammatory disorders and diseases. This drug was much more effective than current NSAIDs . The drug inhibits what are known as transcription factors in RA. The inflammation in the joints in particular may be linked to the production of free oxygen radicals. In addition certain enzymes and Cytokines are released by the inflammatory cells. The compound works by inhibiting key regulatory proteins among which is a prominent one known as NF-kB ; these are also known as transcription factors. Bispan is believed to be very effective in this action. This will not cure **RA**, as is the case for many, but may be much more effective than current NSAIDs.

A new drug called Recently, the FDA approved **Arthotec** by **Searle.** This drug is an improved NSAID that provides significant relief without causing massive GI problems and ulcers. The drug contains misoprostol and diclofenac sodium. The misoprostol reduces the incidence of GI problems ; the diclofenac sodium is enteric coated to lower absorption and irritation to the stomach. If this helps, it is now available.(oxymetholone at 50 mg) has been approved by the FDA for the treatment of anemia.

A new drug, **Anadrol** or oxymetholene has been approved in the US by the FDA. It is ultra important that the doctor and patient be aware that anemia is present in rheumatoid arthritis and inflammatory bowel diseases (also in lupus and cancer and of course aplastic anemia and pernicious anemia, etc. (caution B-12 injections must still be used.) . This work was reported by Dr. Corklin Steinheart, MD and by Unimed Pharmaceuticals. The therapies used to treat diseases such as **RA** (such as gold salts, etc.) as well as the primary disease cause significant anemia. The shortage of red blood cells results in a lack of oxygen transport. If used early, this drug can have a significant good effects on the long term survival of the patient. This medication acts to increase the production of erythropioetin which stimulates red blood cell production; in addition stem cells within the bone marrow also are stimulated to produce red blood cells. It is strongly suggested that **Anadrol** be used with **Methotrexate** and **Folic acid**. This drug, **Anadrol,** is an anabolic steroid and in Category III. The physician is to use care and consult prescription information supplied by Unimed Pharmaceutical. **Of all the medications, this combination may have very dramatic effects for severe RA. It is strongly suggested that his drug combination be used and its efficacy evaluated.**

Recently, the FDA approved **Arthotec** by **Searle.** This drug is an improved NSAID that provides significant relief without causing massive GI problems and ulcers. The drug contains misoprostol and diclofenac sodium. The misoprostol reduces the incidence of GI problems ; the diclofenac sodium is enteric coated to lower absorption and irritation to the stomach. If this helps, it is now available.

Another drug is in massive clinical trials in the US is a COX-2 inhibitor, and may be available by participation in these trials.(See the Appendix for a list of sites.) COX is the enzyme cyclooxygenase that helps to produce prostaglandin's which cause inflammation and pain. COX-1 is OK ,so the drug must only **inhibit COX-2 (COX-2 Inhibitor**). The drug performs this function well and offers a new NSAID that will have few side effects. The current study is funded by Searle and company. Call **214-376-5451,ext 7125** to determine if you will be able to participate in the study. Note: This drug is now approved and available.

There are many other medications under development or currently available in Europe or Canada.

There is a class of drugs which offer real hope of not only treatment but a type of remission . These and other treatments will be described in **Research Frontiers.** Of the work to date, the promise is high **.** There one drug that doesn't have a name yet just a number but offers not only help but a possible complete stoppage of **RA**. Another combination of drugs tried at the Naval Research Institute offers a cure with a one time administration. This work is truly impressive and offers much. Other work involves a vaccine. Unfortunately much of this is in the development stage but much of the work is complete ,and clinical trials should start soon. At the present time, the work by **Cellpro Inc**. can work and may be the front runner as a possible cure (at present).

Chapter 10

Research Frontiers and Advances

Some of the new treatments and advances will be available very soon. One technique that is available **now** is the use of **M**agnetic **R**esonance **I**maging or MRI. This can be used to identify patients with early damage and the progression of the damage. This can be used to help patients with very severe **RA** and in these patients the most powerful combinations of therapies and medicines need to be started early. CT scans or 3D High Resolution X -Rays are also useful for this. The proper use of MRI and high resolution images enables your physician to more accurately treat and evaluate the progress of the disease and the therapy used. Most doctors in the U.S. do not use this since the cost is high ; you have the right to request such treatment and to petition your insurance carrier for payment of MRI.

Cytokine modulators such as **Tenidap** by Pfizer are ready for use and are currently approved in Europe. The current thinking is to actively monitor the patient and use the big guns early in the battle to minimize the damage that can be done. The therapies and the medicines under development will be covered in detail later. This section will cover some of the advances. The details of the research will require some understanding of Immunology which will be explained in a manner such that the average person with some perseverance can understand the basics. The descriptions in this area will not require any detailed medical knowledge and may be easily understood.

Remember the drug **Thalidomide,** and the horrible birth defects that resulted from its use. Obviously the drug was causing genetic mutations. Bad, but only if you are a pregnant mother. If you are post menopausal ,or above about 45 years of age ,and have **RA** or some other Immune disorder this may be what will help. If you are looking for compounds that may help look into drugs that **<u>do</u>** cause birth defects. Look at **drugs that control cancers**; look at **drugs that control AIDS**; look at **drugs used for control of transplant rejection**, etc. There are very good reasons for these statements ,and later this will be explained. This was very obvious to the researchers, and this is exactly what was done and has been done. The **Celgene Corporation** has done experimentation and has developed modified thalidomide that has very useful properties for modulating inflammatory diseases such as **RA**. The work is reported in the *Journal of Medical Chemistry* in the August 1996 issue. This category of compounds even has a new name. The name of the modified thalidomide is **SelCID** (US trademark) . The responsible persons are Dr. Sol Barer (CEO) of **Celgene** and Dr. David Sterling (VP), also with **Celgene**. The drug has the ability to inhibit the overproduction of TNF-a (a Cytokine overproduced by immune cells such as those in a person with **RA** or MS and other diseases.). The drug, **SelCID,** is said to 500 time more potent than **Thalidomide** for this purpose. Patents have been applied for. The release date for this drug is unknown since it must undergo several phases of clinical trials. According to *ABC News* the drug also has the name **Synovir** and has been approved for inflammation from Leprosy . The use is banned for mothers or would be mothers. Physicians will be required to undergo extensive education before being allowed to write prescriptions. Nothing new, doctors are always aware of the dangers and act responsibly. Let us hope that the FDA also acts, since people are suffering (and worse), and need medicines that will work.

Anergen Technology has developed a potent therapy for RA. This was reported in the June 1997 issue of ***Arthritis and Rheumatism*** (USA). One of the compound is called **HC gp-39** . The HC designation infers from Human Cartilage. **HC gp-39** is a protein with a peptide that is recognized by T cells from **RA** patients. The peptide and protein have the capability of blocking the **RA** response to antigens (foreign bodies that with the **RA** patient may be confused with **Self**). This has also been done previously with chicken protein from the sternum area of a baby chicken.

The work done by **IDEC Pharmaceuticals** and **Smith Kline Beecham** was released in late October of 1996. They have a compound called **IDEC-CE9.1/SB 210396.** This may have a name by now. The work was announced by Dr. Craig Wiesenhutter at the Conference of the *American College of Rheumatology, 1996.* The compound is a non-depleting anti-CD4 monoclonal antibody .The antibodies are the result of genetic engineering to produce structural similarity to human (Primate) antibodies. The compound binds to the CD4 protein on helper T cells on RA patients. This action by the antibody reduces the T cell activity and immune responses that are unwanted in RA patients. Thus the disorder and destruction it causes is slowed (but not cured). This shows great promise and may be administered in a doctors office. Hopefully the compound will have a name soon and be start a third phase or later of clinical trials.

A similar effort is reported in *The Journal of Autoimmunity* in 1997, Feb **10:1** 87-97 by P.A. van der Lubbe and coworkers at Leiden Hospital in the Netherlands. They used CD4 monoclonal antibody to treat patients with **RA** . The chimeric monoclonal antibody is called cM-T412 . This type of treatment is also used for certain cancers. The result of the treatment was that the CD4+ and CD45RA+ T cell count decreased dramatically. This reduced inflammation from the attack of the **ABI** on the joints and connective tissue. This treatment is still under investigation.

Medarex announced a new drug for the treatment of immune disorders such as **RA**, Lupus, and ITP (idiopathic thromocytopenia purpura). The work was done with **Ceteon LLC**. The work was described by Dr. Randell T. Curnow of **Medarex** in the 5 Th. *International Bispecific Antibody Conference*. The drug has a designation only of **MDX-33** at present. The drug has the ability to modulate the FcyRI receptor on Immune killer cells . Thus, the bad stuff done by the **Army of the Berserk Immune System** can be stopped or at least slowed. Hopefully this work will move into advanced clinical trials and the drug will acquire a name.

There are vaccines being developed for **RA**. (**This approach offers not only help but potential cures- you can be vaccinated and not acquire RA**). One is by a research team from Jefferson Medical College headed by Dr. J. Bruce Smith. The study was published in the US *Journal of Rheumatology* in March, 1996. The vaccine is comprised of mononuclear white cells that were derived from pregnant women. It is known that pregnancy induces remission in **RA** and that the immune system produces special Cytokines that protect the fetus from attack by the **Army of the Berserk Immune**. The vaccine improves the **RA** and induces the **RA** patient to produce protective Cytokines. This study has had very limited clinical trials. There is another vaccine under study by JHU. This is a vaccine developed by the **Immune Response Corporation**. JHU was actively recruiting volunteers for this study which started in early 1996. The study may be over, but there is a number that can reached for information. Call **410-550-2629** and ask for Mary Bardman. There may be new studies that are in planning that **RA** patients may apply for. The vaccine by **Immune Response** consists of synthetic peptides that shut down specific T cells in an RA patient. Thus, the attack by the **Army of the Berserk Immune** is stopped and tissue damage is averted. This vaccine also has no name at present.

Another study by doctors at the Jefferson Medical College report that the use of injected white blood cells (WBC) from spouses or special individuals was very effective in providing significant improvement in **RA**. The work is reported by Dr. Ginsberg and Dr. Thoburn of the *American College of Rheumatology* (ACR). The theory is that in pregnancy that the fetal cells challenge the maternal immune system. This results in a remission of **RA.** Thus, foreign WBCs from a donor could induce improvement in nonpregnant patients with **RA**. Further information may be obtained from the ACR. Also consult the February issue of the *Journal of Rheumatology*.

In the arena of old stuff modified and retried is a study by the NIH. This is intravenous dioxycycline for RA. The NIH at Warren Grant Magnuson Clinical center is recruiting patients for the study. The recruitment started in June/July of 1997. This works quite well for mild **RA and has no effect on severe RA.**

Auto Immune Inc. has a number of medicines under development. One of the treatments is called **Colloral**. This and other drugs by the same company have proved to be of value for **RA**. The mechanism of action is not reported. The drug has been found to be safe and well tolerated. It is intended as a replacement for patients intolerant of drugs such as **Methotrexate (Golden Boy).**

Another drug is due for release in about 1-2 years (Now available). This is called **Arthotec** and is available currently in at least 27-30 countries. It is a combination of a NSAID diclofenac and misoprostol. Basically it is a NSAID with reduced side effects. This very important issue since gastric and intestinal damage can be very damaging to the patients well being and survival. Recently, the FDA approved **Arthotec** by **Searle.** The misoprostol reduces the incidence of GI problems ; the diclofenac sodium is enteric coated to lower absorption and irritation to the stomach. If this helps, it is **now available**.

Recently , a Boston Life Sciences announced that it will be completing tests of a gene that controls apoptosis or programmed cell death in T-cells. The gene is called BClx-gamma and has been reported in the Journal *Immunity* (in Vol. 7, pp. 629-639, 1997) by Dr. Harvey Cantor of Harvard Medical School. By inhibiting BClx-gamma after T cells are activated, the T cells apoptose and the immune response from the T cells activated in Autoimmunity are suppressed. This work is currently under study and has great promise.

Many new drugs are available in Europe, Canada, and Mexico. For some unknown reason, The FDA requires that a drug that has passed all of the clinical trials be retested in the US. The tests are almost exactly the same as those in Europe and Canada. **Why is this being done** ? The net result is that about 4-5 additional years pass before the patient has access to a **previously proven remedy**. For an **RA** patient, **this is totally unacceptable**. (**This is changing**.) The change is occurring now and is dramatic. Physicians and patients be aware that much medication is now more quickly available.

Chapter 11
THE TOWER OF HOPE

THE US NAVY JOINS IN THE ATTACK

The Navy is on the attack on the **ABI.** Dr. David Harlan, Dr. Allan Kirk, and many other **Naval Research Institute** Researchers as well as Researchers from the **University of Wisconsin**, and Scientists from **Biogen** and **Genetics Institute of Cambridge** announced the results of pioneering work on a technique to prevent the rejection of transplants. The work is specifically aimed for mismatched organ transplantation. The work was announced on *ABC News' Good Morning America* ,and in an article in the August 5, 1997 Issue of the *Proceedings of the National Academy of Science.* The technique is novel and uses some very basic mechanisms . T cells operate in pairs. One does the basic determination that the foreign material (cell, antigen, etc.) is foreign ,and another helper T cell verifies the antigen and calls to the rest of the Immune System to mount an attack on the foreign antigen (may be a transplant but also may be **Self**). Thus, the transplanted organ is attacked unless drugs are used to suppress the response. However, it is possible to stop this reaction. This is done with **CTLA4-Ig** (a B-7 specific fusion protein) and **anti-CD40 ligand (CD40L-5C8),** a very specific monoclonal antibody)**.** The combination of the fusion protein and the antibody was effective in preventing the costimualtion of the T cells that provide alarm to the Immune System. The combination of the two compounds serves to educate the T cells. Thus, the process is used for a brief period only, without the need for extended application as is now the case with immunospressive drugs that must be taken for life. For simplicity, the fusion protein and the specific antibody have educated the T cells that the transplanted organ is to be treated as **Self.** Thus, for other immune disorders where **Self** is not recognized by the Immune System; the response may be altered and the Immune attack stopped and the alarm and cascade process is stopped by chemical reeducation of the T cells . Thus , potentially, **RA, Lupus**, and **MS** could be altered in a profound manner. The technique is also non toxic and long lasting. This work ,and work similar to this, is the **New Hope** and that hope is **very promising**. The work has only been done on basic primates to date, but human trials must be planned and if successful, the **Magic Gate** is opened and **Hope is Transformed to An Effective Treatment** for transplant organ rejection, **RA, Lupus**, and **MS**.

The Big Guns of the Navy bequeath Hope for the Future in Abundance. I feel that this course of Research should be very productive and produce effective treatments. It may not be today, but not too long from now. The Navy and the Country must have immense pride in these people. Of all the work done by the dedicated researchers and Doctors, this is a **very real hope** and may be part of the future for the treatment of **RA.**

VERY NEW DRUGS UNDER EVALUATION

OXIGENE has two news drugs called **<u>Neu-Sensamide and Oxi-104</u>** that can control inflammation and **Sepsis** (a profound blood borne infection that may result from organ infection as well as the blood- may be **fatal** , about 50% or more mortality). These drugs suppress the release of tumor necrosis factor- α (TNF-α). The control of inflammation is important. **The control of sepsis will control life or death for the patient. Sepsis can be fatal for RA patients** since they are taking or have taken medications that severely depress the immune system. **Thus, when sepsis occurs, they are in <u>Extreme</u> Mortal Danger ,and new treatments such as this may be lifesaving.** Massive antibiotic injection is used ,but may not control other effects of sepsis.

A new drug has been developed and has approval by the FDA. This drug is called **Anzemet** and is the product of **Hoechst Marion Rouse** . This drug effectively controls the nausea effects of chemotherapy drugs. Thus **RA** patient taking **Imuran** etc. that have problems with severe nausea can have relief and the benefits of the **Imuran** etc. This may sound trivial but the nausea can be so severe that some patients will **stop** taking the medication. This presents a real problem since the disease (disorder) has progressed to the point where these medications are needed. Thus, **Anzemet is <u>extremely</u> important when using Imuran.**

Roche has a new drug for transplants that may rival cyclosporine for transplant patients. The drug is called **Zenapax** and may have use for severe **RA.** The drug not only has a name but has passed rigorous tests and is in Phase III trials. It is designed for renal transplants and the transplant rejection. **Zenapax** has recently been granted approval by the FDA Biological Response Modifier Committee. It is approved for the use of the use of patient having problems with renal transplants. It is now under investigation for other autoimmune problems. The drug called **Zenapax** ® is also known as daclizumab. The FDA Biological Response Modifier Committee has now recommended approval. It is extremely effective in reducing organ graft survival such as kidneys. It is **safe** and **highly effective**. It is believed that it will ,or will be very effective in treating other autoimmune diseases. The compound works by binding to a highly active receptor on the activated T cell and suppressing the action of the T cell that would normally result in the destruction of the transplanted organ. Thus, it succeeds in stopping the autoimmune reaction. The action is from the binding of IL-2 to the high affinity IL-2 receptor on the

T cell. As contrasted with more conventional treatments such as cyclosporine , there were **no** significant adverse side effects of the medicine. These results were presented to the *American Society of Transplant Physicians* in May of 1996 by Dr. Kirk . The principal investigator is Dr. Flavio Vincenti, Professor of Clinical Medicine at the University of California at San Francisco. Dr. Flavio Vincenti is currently studying the use of **Zenapax** ® for patients with autoimmune disease such as **RA**. As of December, 1997, the drug is now available in the US. Additional studies are reported in the *New England Journal of Medicine.*

One of the frontiers of **RA** research is genetic manipulation (therapy). This is being actively done in Japan and Europe on humans with success. Gene transfer and surgery are used concurrently ,and are very successful. One therapy is the introduction of an anti-arthritis protein into a joint directly. This will result in a protein product that reproduces itself and will transfer to other joints. Thus there is no need for additional injection, etc. The anti-arthritic protein (one of many) is called an Interlukein-1 receptor antagonist. This work bears careful scrutiny as to the vast improvements that it offers. This type of therapy where the genetic information is altered or the path is changed should be very fruitful with great potential for the **RA** patient and for other autoimmune disorders.

The **Weizman Institute** reports that the immune response can be controlled by a molecule called **NF-kappaB. NF-kappa** is regulated by the inhibition effects of **IkappaB.** Researchers at the Institute report that this process is initiated by the activation of **NIK** protein which they have cloned in genetic experiments. Their research is exploring potential therapeutic targets of the immune system. The technology ,which is very much still in the research stage, offers the potential for either development of blocking effects for autoimmune disease or enhancement effects for immune depression such as AIDS and other diseases. This work offers great promise.

Recently researchers have discovered a gene usually present only in cancerous cells. This was reported at the Nov.12, 1997 meeting of *the American College Of Rheumatology.* A more complete description may be obtained from the *Proceedings* and the *Journal Of Rheumatology.* The work is headed by Dr. Gary Firestein of the University of California-San Diego School of Medicine. The defects are seen in a gene called p53. This gene normally monitors cell characteristics and conveys molecular messages as to the fate of damaged cells. This gene, when defective, also has a major causative role in cancer. Dr. Firestein found this gene in the synovium of **RA** patients. Thus, the normal function of the gene is rendered useless ,and the **RA** becomes more aggressive in the synovial area and readily destroys the joint and bone. A complete description of the process may be found in the Sept. 30, 1997 issue of *The Proceedings of The National Academy of Science*. This is an important clue as to the nature of the causative factors for the disease.

The **Big Guns of the US Naval Research Institute** are exploring reeducation of the immune system-**it works folks** ! **ProCell** and others have perfected stem cell replacement-a drastic procedure but-**it works folks, AND IS CURRENTLY AVAILIABLE !** The genetic approach works and is under investigation-preliminary reports are that it too **works for RA** and other autoimmune diseases and immune deficiency diseases as well. There is more good news: The drug approval process in the US is being streamlined and improved. It is hoped that the bill makes its way out of Congress and is approved.

New and Real Help from Congress

The new bill in Congress (105 Congress) is known as The Drug and Biological Reform Act of 1997, and is currently assigned as H.R. 1411. The sponsor is Rep. Burr and the Bill was introduced on 4/23/97. The bill greatly reforms and speeds the process of Drug approval. The most important provision is Section 25. Here there is a process that will enable you expanded access to unapproved therapies. This procedure will allow the physician access to new medicines and drugs under evaluation ,and if certain conditions are met, the doctor is allowed to access and use Investigational Drugs. This section and other key sections are included in the Appendix. **This bill is extremely important** and deserves full support. The doctor does not have to enter the drug Investigational protocol ,but he does have to met specific criteria. For patients with diseases or conditions that have no comparable therapy and have exhausted all means of treatment, and the risk of using the drug (s) is not greater than the risk of the disease, then that physician may have access to the Investigational Drug or Treatment. Thus, many of the drugs and treatments mentioned will be accessible if the bill is passed and the criteria are satisfied. If this is true, then the statement : " **I have no more medications or procedures that can be tried** " **WILL NEVER BE APPROPRIATE.** Thus, the **Platitude song** will **not** be on the TOP 40 any more. A new song will be repeated and sung with great enthusiasm.

I have walked in the Garden and have seen the Light-
Yours is a Case that I can Right.

And, to be Sung Over and Over to All Who Suffer and Seek Help

All will soon learn this simple song.

The bill in its Senate version (S830) passed and was signed into law by the President. A summary is included in Appendix C. Public Law: 105-115 (11/21/97) SPONSOR: Senator Jeffords (introduced 06/05/97) A short excerpt from the law is included here.

(Sec. 104) Authorizes the Secretary of Health and Human Services to authorize the shipment of Investigational drugs for the diagnosis or treatment of a serious disease or condition in emergency situations.

Authorizes any person, through a licensed physician, to request, and any manufacturer or distributor to provide to the physician, such a drug if specified requirements are met.

Directs the Secretary, after submission of a protocol intended to provide widespread access, to permit expanded access under a treatment Investigational new drug (IND) application if certain requirements are met.

The law has teeth as well. Consider this:

(Sec. 106) Amends the FDCA to allow a manufacturer, in certain circumstances, to disseminate to health care practitioners, pharmacy benefit managers, health insurance insurers, group health plans, or government agencies certain information on the safety, effectiveness, or benefit of a use not described in the approved labeling of a drug if the manufacturer meets certain requirements. Allows the Secretary, on ordering a manufacturer to cease dissemination, to order the manufacturer to correct information that has been disseminated. Makes failure to comply with this section a prohibited act. Terminates the effectiveness of the amendments made by this section on a specified date.

This is major progress in the battle to save the suffering. Congress and the President Clinton deserve overwhelming praise.

Chapter 12
POSSIBLE CAUSES OF RA

The exact cause of **RA** is unknown. **At least the true and exact cause is unknown**. Many theories abound as to why the disease occurs. The leading theories are genetic, endocrine, and infections (viral or bacterial or both) and/or combinations of these that lead to **RA**. This section will examine some of these, and explore possible other causes or related causes. Basically, the Immune System loses its ability to recognize Self and attacks Self with a vengeance that causes great damage and eventual destruction of Self. I have used the term Army of the Berserk Immune or **ABI.** This ,of course is not scientific, but in order to be understandable some of the terminology needs to be simplified. This is not a simple task since the Immune System is **exceedingly complex** and actually elegant in its mechanisms, etc. It is so profound in its inception ,and has so many safeguards that one is almost driven to look for a foreign antigen trigger possibly with a slight genetic defect combined.

All the explanations lack a solid foundation and await significant research. The approach of reeducation such as that by the Naval Research Institute is very promising since it has as a given that the Immune System will attack a transplant organ or in the case of **RA** will attack self. Thus, the approach is to reeducate the system with the proper compounds and procedures. This is normally done by the body itself in the bone marrow and in the Thymus. The other approach by ProCell Inc. is just as effective , but involves considerable expense ,and may not be applied if the disease is too far advanced. However, this case is rare-it should work for almost all. The only problem may be the insurance companies; once the procedure is widely accepted, this should not be a problem.

There are some real clues that may prove productive. Lyme disease is carried by Deer ticks and the Lyme bacillus. In addition to having Lyme disease, you have **RA** and in the past the true disease was not detected until considerable damage had been done. The flagellum protein is a clone or close copy of the body's own protein in the axon. Thus, in the process of the normal response to the antigen, the Immune System attacks self since part of the attacker antigen is almost the same as Self. Thus the immune system is not berserk but doing its job; the real problem here is that the attacker is a copy of parts of Self. Thus in addition to **RA**, Lyme disease will cause nerve damage. Fortunately the disease is effectively treated with antibiotics. Thus the Lyme disease and the pseudo **RA** is cured (sometimes).

Some recent work suggests that an AIDS like virus can trigger or simulate Lupus, **RA**, and at least two other autoimmune diseases. Again, there is no inherent defect in the Immune System; it is attacking an antigen that is part of Self. In scanning the literature, I was greatly impressed how therapies for AIDS usually had a profound beneficial effect on **RA** patients. There was a small research group in Bath, England, that for years used a combination of thalidomide and AIDS drugs on **RA** patients and had <u>remarkable success</u> in treating the **RA**. The AIDS patient with **RA** did not have his prime disease cured ,but if he had concurrent **RA**, it was brought under control.

The autoimmune disease is almost always linked to a particular class of antigens. The most common is called HLA and a type II relation will result in **RA**. Different classes of antigens and the reaction to these lead to various autoimmune responses. Thus, the genetic trigger emerges. The link is most strong for HLA-B27 antigen and **RA** and Lupus. This can be detected by tests and has been done at JHU for years. The other clue is a strong response to Penicillamine at first with the response quickly disappearing. This is also an indication of severe **RA**.

A certain hepatitis and billary cirrhosis overlap and result in autoimmune disease such as **RA** and Lupus. See *Lancet* 1:292, 1987 and *Western Journal of Medicine* 153: 439,1990 for more complete and meaningful descriptions. Thus, the link is very strong that the Immune System is essentially OK and attacking something that is not being detected unless it causes known malfunctions such as Liver disease or the well known effects of Lyme disease. A burning question arises as to why the AIDS drugs have such a profound effect. **Is suppression of the Immune System correct ? Are symptoms being treated and not the true cause ?** Can a bacterium or virus be present that is not detected since it closely resembles Self ? Is it possible that an antigen stimulates a response, and then when tests are made, the virus or bacterium is gone but the response to it is still active ?

Tests are now underway to treat the **RA** and similar autoimmune responses by feeding the autoantigen to the patient. If type II collagen (from the sternum of baby chickens) is given to patients with **RA** , remarkable improvement is noted. If cow myelin protein is given to MS patients, they improve.. It appears that the current medications can only control and NEVER cure the **RA** and the like. The ability to control is dubious. It may be that there is nothing wrong with the Immune System and all that is being done is the treatment of symptoms-**Poor Procedure** ! Of course, if this is all that the patient can get, then that is what they will get (unfortunately).

The book by Henry Schammel " *The Arthritis Breakthrough* " published by M. Evans, New York, 1993 promises much. In the book the role of the mycoplasma and **RA** is explored at great length. The cause of RA is postulated to be the "viral cousin " of the causative virus against which the Immune System generates antibodies. The treatment proposed is the monocycline version of tetracycline . This appears to be valid if the **RA is mild** and treated early. Thus, the idea that the Immune System is OK basically may be valid for mild **RA**. This lack of a distinction may be important and severe **RA** may appear to be the same as the mild or versions resulting from such as Lyme bacilli or virus like mycoplasma. Near the end of the book the observation is made about patients with AIDS and **RA**; the **RA** disappears in some cases. Again, the connection between some forms of **RA** and infectious agents may be well established in the thought process of some; however, I do not believe that this is a universal phenomena.

Another observation is that persons with severe intestinal permeability and those with intestinal obstructions, plus a genetic defect or predisposition may develop **RA**. In patients that were overtly obese and used an intestinal shunt to limit the amount of nutrient's that could be absorbed, there were some very interesting results other than the loss of body mass. Some shunts produced a blockage effect that resulted in some continuous accumulation. **All** of those patients developed **RA**. I don't see the connection but the probability was 100% . Thus a combination of genetics and an intestinal problem could have a significant causal effect. **Anna** had a so called intestinal crimp or blockage that caused her severe problems. Her doctors should have removed this when she was a child. In addition her mother died of cancer when she was in her early forties-about the same time of life (40-45) that **Anna contracted RA.** It is shown in the literature that if you are female ,you are three times more likely to have or contract **RA** than a male, and this has the greatest statistical probability of occurrence just about 40-45 years of age. Concurrent exposure to some unknown antigen also may help to trigger the process.

Textbook explanations range from unknown to some postulates. Some mention endocrine con - committal factors. Some talk of unknown viral or genetic triggers. Of course all are postulates and await more study.

Still in the Research Lab

Benjamin Segal and coworkers report in *The Journal Of Immunology* (Vol. 158,No. 11 Issue 06-01-97) that microbial products , bacterial DNA, and the like can induce an autoimmune response. Other researchers have observed similar phenomena. Another study implicated the same component as promoting the Immune response. A study by Schimmer and coworkers in the same *Journal Of Immunology* (Volume 159 Number 8) implicates streptococcal wall substance as readily inducing immune arthritis. Many other studies can be found that implicate some common or uncommon bacillus or virus. Thus, the postulate the immune response is linked to a real antigen appears to be valid.

There a multitude of studies underway and some should be very definitive. Another approach is to correct the disease early in its inception. The body has an organs specially designed to do this such as the Thymus. One study (of many) by Charles Egwuagu and coworkers explores the role of thymic expression on autoimmune disease. This may be found in *The Journal of Immunology* , Vol. 159, No. 7 Issue of 10-01-97. Here a detailed study is made of the role of the Thymus in correction and development of resistance to autoimmune disease. Could it be possible that any treatment that stimulates thymic activity could help ? The answer awaits.

The Thymus

The Thymus plays a very important role in immune response. T cells develop here and learn to be able to differentiate between Self and non-Self. This process is very strong in early childhood unless the patient has DiGeorges syndrome. Sometime after puberty, the Thymus becomes much smaller ,but is believed to be still active. The treatment for this syndrome is a 10% solution of calcium gluconate . The next step is the transplant of fetal Thymic tissue. One wonders if this would help **RA**. Since the Thymus is the great educator of T cells, would not its restoration at least help? The thymus can be helped by vitamin C, E, B6, zinc, and selenium. The use of thymic hormones may be helpful. It is reported that oral bovine thymus concentrates do help. As a matter of fact, AIDS therapy includes such and it has been noted previously that there is a strong therapy link between autoimmune and immune deficiency diseases.

The thymus extract should be used for at least three months to achieve help. The daily dose should be about 120 mg EQ. of pure polypeptide or 500 mg of the crude polypeptide. This may not cure or appear to offer massive relief , but it may help.

A possible treatment would be to extract some of the thymus of the patient and grow the cells to a certain mass and reintroduce these thymic cells to the patient. If supplemented by growth hormones, this should (may) help.

One other compound that can be obtained over the counter is **DHEA** . This is currently under investigation for Lupus but may also be effective for RA. **DHEA** is a natural hormone produced by the adrenal glands; it is currently available as a nutritional supplement and requires no prescription. The FDA is considering changing this ,and this compound become available only through prescription. This may not happen but since good results are being obtained, some of the drug manufacturers want its status changed ; at least the version that they will be making.

A Possible Cause of Rheumatoid Arthritis (RA)

The true cause of RA is unknown, but this is the hypothesis that I think may have some validity. First you must have a specific genetic marker or the like or predisposition to the condition. These markers are discussed in the literature as alterations to the surface of the lymphocyte . These genetic effects have well defined structure and have very specific names. (See Appendix and References). This may make the probability of acquiring the disorder more pronounced but may not be a 100% causal factor. To wit, it is possible to not have the genetic effect or defect ,and still acquire the disorder ; however, it is more likely that if you do have the marker, the probability is higher. The disease may be caused by a mutant or variant of a very common pathogen such as some species of streptococci or some bacterium or possibly some virus. The Immune System mounts an attack against the antigen. The initial symptoms may range from unnoticeable to severe. These do not last. The invader is either destroyed or if a virus, it is part of some cellular structure. The unique characteristic of the antigen is that it closely resembles or is able to appear as a close relative or imitation of self. The response of the Immune System will be variable. Most will be able to make the distinction and the response will be mild and quickly over. Others will have a severe response and the episode will also be quickly over. Some will have a response that is confused or massive and continues long after the antigen is destroyed. Since the molecular response is patterned; parts of self are now targets. The Immune System continues its attack on those cells of Self that it perceived on a molecular basis to be foreign antigens. Thus the disease starts. The response may be to a true virus such as a mycoplasma or some other infective agent. These organism can be destroyed and treated and antibiotics are effective. Other forms of the disease are mild but are unaffected by antibiotics, but are affected by such as Penicillamine and the like. In other cases where the Immune System responds as if a foreign army had invaded the body, the response is massive and continuous. This form of the disease or disorder responds at first to the likes of Penicillamine but after a short period of time, this has no effect or minimal effect. The antigen can never be found since the Immune System destroyed it long ago, but the molecular imitation of the antigen was such that Self is also included in the attack. This will continue indefinitely, and may be reinforced. Thus a partial relapse or vast improvement may be noted. However, the antigen is still around and continuously attacks; the remission does not last since the Immune System remounts its attack and the disease restarts with a vengeance. This called a flare and is merely a repetition of the start of the disease. Careful monitoring of the patient would reveal the source antigen. This will require blood samples to be taken daily, and analyzed for a period of about 6 months to as much as a year. This may or may not be successful. If a virus, the antigen may have such an effective hiding ability in the hosts cells that detection is very difficult. Thus, a better procedure would be to use mice, and do the tests before the disease started and in an accelerated fashion. This type of work may be underway and possible antigens may have been identified. I hope this is the case. The only truly effective treatment for the severe form of **RA** is reeducation of the Immune System such as being done by the Navy and others or total stem cell replacement. Other therapies that currently exist can, at best, only control the progress of the disease. For mild **RA** almost any therapy works and rightfully so since the Immune System response is always mild. If the antigens or antigens can be identified, then suitable vaccines can be developed. This would totally eradicate this disease; all or those with the genetic markers would be vaccinated. The attention of the researchers could be diverted to other diseases of which there are many. Of course, this may not be the path or may not be how the disease is started but it is a path and needs investigation by serious professionals.

The list of infection related arthritis is large on a comparative basis. In addition to Lyme induced arthritis are many more. Gonococcus from Gonorrhea spreads from the genitals to the joints. This can be effectively treated with antibiotics. The effectiveness of the treatment is related to the therapy and the active presence of the bacilli. Streptococcal infection can induce damage to the heart. This is sort of a roaming arthritis and is usually well treated with antibiotics. This is known as Rheumatic fever and is very rare in the US in the present time. Arthritis may also be associated with HIV virus. This is usually not severe and may be effectively treated with NSAIDs which of course have no effect on the AIDS. Viral arthritis is rare and usually stops as the viral infection is cured or the Immune System stops the virus on its own.

Reactive arthritis also known as Reiter's syndrome can result from a severe bowel or urinary tract infection. This too responds well to therapy and normally does not progress. This occurs in those with the well known genetic marker HLA-B27. Other very rare causes are fungi and other virus but all are mild and respond to therapy. The cause of reactive arthritis is unknown, and it does not respond as to antibiotics as the other forms of infection induced or associative arthritis.

RA acts like the patient has the flu or some other microbe such as some form of bacilli. Yet none can be found. The only other form of arthritis that has as similar profile is Reactive or Reiter's syndrome. Both have genetic predisposition. The exact genetic defect for **RA** may be similar but it also may not. The genetic marker sometimes found in those with **RA** is HLA-DR4. Thus the true cause of **RA** is a real mystery.

There are many diseases for which the exact cause is not known but the treatment is reasonably effective. In the case of the mild **RA** or the forms just discussed, this is true. For severe **,** only very toxic medications have much effect after about 3 years or less. The best that can be done at present is the Bone Marrow Transplantation as done by **ProCell** and others.

Anna's Story Continues.......

The engine roared as if it had a life of its own. The sound was deafening and definitely primitive. Smoke ,oil, and -the smell- truly exhilarating. The propeller was increasing in speed and generating a wind such that never seemed possible. Everything shook and vibrated-even us. The power of the old Pratt & Whitney Radial was an experience that few humans could ever forget- it permeates your senses- you feel the power of the machine-you feel the power yourself. I can fly-no question about it. The grass is against the ground as you view your feet; the cables move, the whole scene is as if you were encased and part of some primitive being. The tension mounts- the beast bumps along the grass with continually increasing speed-the wind -the wind literally has a life of its own, and you feel part of it. The craft leaves the earth suddenly; birds quickly move, the clouds beckon. You are now part of the air; the wires between the wings hum. Your soul-your very being soars as the craft lifts you to higher and higher heights; the clouds are very close now. You can feel the moisture-the craft hums; it is alive. You and the pilot and your Love know that- the world is below-there is no room for mortals. We are now part of the heavens and look down on what we once were. We roll, we lift still further- your very soul sings. Flight is possible-you are part of the heavens-the birds are now beside and beneath you. The sun-the sun shines ever so brightly. It is almost impossible to believe that the light could be so bright. The craft turns and lifts again; you feel heavy as the acceleration is felt by your being. Such is a Sunday afternoon at the aerodrome in the Magic Kingdom.

Once back on tera-firma, you feel a little bit shaken, but at the same time your being is till soaring. The experience provided by biplanes and aircraft from an earlier age enables one to understand why there is such a love of the aircraft. Anna loved these planes and we made many a Sunday afternoon an experience usually reserved only for the Angels. Our love soared to the same heights ,and we also flew as surely as the aircraft. The range of people at the aerodrome in the Magic Kingdom was astounding; a Minister from a local church was an avid enthusiast. He ,with the help of others, had completely restored a very- very old Sopwith Camel . The craft was a work of art as well as engineering; it had a very distinct personality that called to you from its glorious past. Some think machines are machines and that is that. Of course they are machines ,but they stimulate a primitive and an unknown part of our being that some never know even exists. It does exist-it just needs the proper stimulus.

Stand behind or close to an older car from the 60's with some phenomenal engine that engulfs you with the staccato of its power as it springs to life. The purr of its engine is a majestic sound that breathes life- a life that may not be familiar, but a being nevertheless . Machines of course are machines ,but they can inspire -the process of creating such and bringing them to life is an experience that few would ever forget or would want to forget. The strong cry of a healthy baby and the purr that emanates, as it is encompassed by its mother, in an embrace, is of the purest form of love and the eminence of such. It is a feeling that is strongly conveyed to your higher being; you feel the love, the power of each. The love from the baby, and that of the mother toward the baby are truly divine. Machines ,of course , are machines but when created with love, that love emendates, and encircles you as the device sings it own song- we are reminded in our being of strong emotions enhanced by the song of Being. I am that I am- **Listen** and look around**;** there are many such songs.

Life was Good with Anna

"Shall I compare thee to a summer's day?
Thou art more lovely and more temperate:
Rough winds do shake the darling buds of May,
And summer's lease hath all too short a date:
Sometime too hot the eye of heaven shines,
And often is his gold complexion dimmed;
And every fair from fair sometime declines,
By chance or nature's changing course untrimmed;
But thy eternal summer shall not fade
Nor lose possession of that fair Thou owest;
Nor shall Death brag Thou wander'st in his shade,
When in eternal lines to time Thou growest:
So long as men can breathe or eyes can see,
So long lives this and this gives life to thee. "

Sonnet XVIII (William Shakespeare)

Anna had two rings that she always wore. One was high purity gold , and was her wedding ring. The other was Sterling silver and was worn on her last index finger. I have been wearing this ring, and some very peculiar transformations have been occurring. The joint has become inflamed. It increased in size from 13 to 17 mm wide and from 14 to 17 mm deep. It has a nodule of sorts on the interior side and was becoming very painful at night. I became so alarmed that I have recently stopped wearing the ring. The inflammation is better and the pain is lessening. There is something in the ring or on its surface that is responsible for this. The other comparable joint is normal as well as all other joints.

When I examine the ring, I notice a slight pitting of the surface on the interior that would be next to the skin. I have considered the alloys that make up Sterling silver and can find no reason for the joint inflammation. The only other possible conclusion is that there is some pathogen in or on the surface that is penetrating the skin and causing the joint inflammation. The little finger has no effective use except for typing and gripping. Thus there is no physical reason for the inflammation. It has happened before, and after I removed the ring, the inflammation got better. Thus, I am led to believe that some bacillus or virus is alive or in a spore form and embedded in the ring's surface. It is possible that his microorganism penetrates the moist skin beneath the ring and causes the inflammation. The organism migrates to the synovial fluid of the joint and is attacked by the Immune System. If there is no genetic marker such as mentioned previously, then only a local inflammation will occur. This has been repeatedly observed. If prone to the genetic defect, this may have progressed to some other condition-maybe; maybe not. The inflammation was so noticeable that it woke me in my sleep. There is something there -it is not simply that the Immune System is causing a local inflammation for no reason whatever. My feeling is that this is something that could be grown in a culture with one of the ingredients for the microbe being synovial fluid. I don't have the equipment, but would suggest that this be done by those proficient in such. It is my belief that you will find some organism that grows in the joint region and is under serious attack by the Immune System. Call it microbe **RAX.** **RAX** lives in pits and crevices of metals that are subjected to warm saline solution and other microorganism commonly found on the skin. It migrates inward and multiplies. The Immune System kills it, and after **RAX** is dead, the attack stops. If the genetic code has suitable coding, the attack progresses ,even after all of the **RAX has been destroyed.** Thus, a person with the defective genetics must be treated promptly with substances that will kill the **RAX,** and restore proper Immune function. It may be some common or uncommon antibiotic that must be injected locally to kill **RAX.** The restoration of the Immune System may done with compounds and approaches as pioneered by the Naval Research Institute. To prevent further occurrence, a proper vaccine must be developed.

I **know** that **RAX** is lurking on the interior surface of this ring. I am afraid to wear it again. The killer has made himself known. My task is to convince persons with the proper equipment to isolate and identify **RAX.** I only have computers, books, and the like. The other key to the puzzle is that the patient will have a very active surface saline that has compounds that will attack inferior metals readily. I greatly fear **RAX-I know it to be a killer.** It is curious that much of the so called treatment for **RA** is to depress the Immune System. **Wrong** approach boys-**you need to reeducate the Immune response and kill the killer. You will never find it since by the time the tests are done, the Immune System has destroyed all of the RAX.** Thus, the organism lurks on the surface of the skin probably borne there by contact. The other necessary ingredient is saline and warmth and perhaps a certain pH range. Thus, the killer has been discovered (A postulate at best- but interesting).

Of course there will be those that will discount the above as the petulations of a bereaved spouse ,and give no credence to the observations made so simply. This could be so ,but then maybe not. It is the interest of all concerned to make the tests. A patient with active severe **RA** must wear a simple silver alloy ring for about 3 months. Examine the surface of the ring. It is my belief that the organism will lurk there . The other necessary tests are genetic typing. I know that his can be done.

I am afraid to wear the ring again. I will keep the ring in a warm environment, but eventually the organism will die and will not be traceable. I could use a sterile cotton swab with a saline (about 0.2%) and rub this across my skin and feed **RAX.** This may keep the organism alive-then again, it may not. The other possibility is that **RAX is alive and well in me.** This bothers me somewhat since the implications are so serious. I will wait and hope that the inflammation goes down.

Anna's Story Continues..........

The stars shine brightly; almost as if one could touch them, yet I know they are thousands of light years away. The slap, slap of the water on the hull and gentle whisper as the air flows over the sails are the only sounds present. The peace and serenity are profound ;I love sailing at night in the summer. The sensation is so relaxing and reaches the very core of your being. You must do this to truly know the experience. Whatever is bothering you will evaporate. Whatever worries you have will cease to exist. You will feel to be apart of nature and all fear will go with the wind. To be effective, no external power is permitted-only the wind. After about two hours or so the feeling of inner peace will appear. Many thoughts will pass and the pleasure will be like none other you may have known. I think fondly of Anna and miss her so.

Recent research points to a possible cause of **RA**, MS, and Lupus. There seems to be some viral agent partly responsible for one of each or all of these disorders. The researchers note a correlation between causative factors for the three disorders. There may be one viral agent ; there may be three. In addition, the patient has to have distinctive genetic markers such as HLA-B27 or HLA-DR4 for **RA** and correspondence for the other disorders such as Lupus and MS. Some believe that the virus may be a variant or mutation of Herpes. Others point to the Epstein-Barr virus, especially for Lupus. Others believe the viral attack to be very slow. The time required to be noticed is from 3-4 months or more and then only locally. **RAX** may be a viral pathogen-only good tests would reveal this; **RAX** may be a combination of viral and bacilli that attack very slowly. It is still a mystery, but I am certain that there is something on the surface of that ring that is a pathogen. After about 3 days of not wearing the ring, the joint is beginning not to hurt and the swelling is going down. I feel that if I had the genetic markers associated with either **RA** or Lupus or MS, that I would be in serious trouble. It is my opinion that the slow viral attack or whatever is the causative plus the secondary factor being genetic. From this and information from researchers, there appears to a similar causal relationship.

In addition, I have a friend that has recently (about one year ago) acquired **RA**. She got the **RA** about 4 months after moving into a recently purchased house that was the former property of a woman with MS. From the limited information and experience that I have ,there appears to be a link. **RAX** or whatever is a common pathogen and lives and grows very slowly. The Immune System of the susceptible may mount a massive counter attack to **RAX** or whatever. The pathogen may closely, on a molecular level, resemble some cell(s) in the host patient. Hence the Immune System continues the attack on itself as well as **RAX**. Three may be three or more variants of **RAX** that in **RA** prefer synovial fluid; in MS prefer outer myelin sheath cell and so on. The semblance may be such that very sophisticated tests would be required to ID the pathogen as opposed to the host cell.

Some researchers have found that by injecting myelin basic protein into the Thymus that some immunity is provided. Could it be that injecting collagen would induce relief in RA- **Bingo !-It does !!!**

Many papers report that a virus ,HHV-6 , may have a distinct cause effect for MS. For a susceptible host, the virus acts like a trigger mechanism. This virus is virtually undetectable and may be dormant for long periods of time. This guy may be a relative of **RAX**; may not. These are important clues and should be vigorously perused. The names are subject to change, and at present may seem almost silly, but we have to start somewhere.

Anna's Story Continues.........

They were just playing a rerun of *American Bandstand* from 1979. The *Village People* sang " YMCA" and "Macho-Macho Man"**. ....** It was a warm night ,and we were all on the dance floor at the Seashore. Our favorite band was singing and playing. It was such fun and we were **SO** HAPPY ! Life flooded around , and everyone near us was having such a good time. The disco music of the 70's-great ,and mostly just fun. The throb and rhythm of the music permeated your being with joy, and dance was something that you <u>had</u> to do. As your body moved to the music your soul sung, and you rejoiced in life ,and, in particular, being able to share life with one of the most warm and loving beings created by God. **Anna** was the very essence of life personified; merely being near her made you happy. It was hard to explain-a force exuded from her that surely was created in Heaven itself. It was not just me that felt this way; everyone that she came in contact with felt the same feeling. You were flooded-overwhelmed with her goodness and being. I never have experienced such since or before. If there had been an Angel created just for us-she was it. The love was a more than an emotion and feeling and all enjoyed it.

" Hay-Hay, I'm going to be a Macho Man-Hey, Hey Hey ! " The Village people loudly sung. That was one night of many. The stars twinkled and the Moon smiled ; I could even hear the Angels singing the song-there was such goodness and love and warmth. **Love** Itself was in our midst and we all felt it.

Chapter 13

God and His Angels Intervene

It is very quiet now- I can even hear the clock tick. This is quite unusual since this clock is very very quiet but the silence strongly pervades all :

" **T**he gingham dog and the calico cat
Side by side on the table sat;
'Twas half past twelve, and (what do you think !)
Nor one nor t'other had slept a wink !
…………………..
Next morning, where the two had sat !
They found no trace of dog or cat;

And some folks think unto this day
That burglars stole that pair away !

But the truth about the cat and pup

Is this: **They ate each other up !**
Now, what do you think of that ! "

The Duel by Eugene Field (1850-1895) (slightly abridged)

Just before Anna died, her cat ,Tut, died. The Vet said it was some mysterious illness that only rarely affects cats, but I know better. He was leaving to be with Anna-he knew more than we. **There is a special place where they both shall be and romp and play with Glee . And how do I know all this - "*I don't fancy or exaggerate-I got my news from the Chinese plate!*" Thus was this and that was that ,and you must believe all for I do not exaggerate !**

Crohn's Disease

In addition to all her problems with **RA**, Anna had Crohn's disease as well. It wasn't clear just when it was acquired, but it made it presence known with deadly fury. She lost almost 3 pints of blood before the doctors could operate ,and the extent of the disease was greater than originally thought. I am thankful she had a fabulous surgeon- he saved her life.

Crohn's disease is an inflammation of the lower intestines causing ulceration in both the large and small intestines. Sometimes this effect makes its diagnosis difficult since it may appear to be ulcerative colitis, but this is not the case. The other key difference is that the damage the intestines is inclusive not just interior or superficial. The greatest damage is to the lower end of the small intestine just as it empties to the large intestine. This defect has to be removed surgically and a small incision is made in the wall of the abdomen ,and the stoma is brought out. The operation is called an Illeostomoy and the stoma is fitted with an Ostomy appliance to capture the discharge from the intestine. The major problem is that the mechanism that caused the problem is still active and a future occurrence is likely. This happened again about three years later and the operation had to be repeated (twice).

The cause of Crohn' disease is unknown. Some theories relate the cause to an abnormal response of the Immune System to some pathogen in the contents of the bowl. One recent observation is that a certain genetic marker is usually found in patients with this disease . The same medicines used to treat **RA** are used to treat or alleviate Crohn's disease. Of these , recently, Methotrexate and cyclosporine have found to be very effective (Curious!). If one looks in medical texts, especially British, the active role of the cells of the small intestine are well explained. These are active parts of the Immune System ,and play a not too well defined role in the management and control of T cells that are supposed to immunologically competent lymphocytes after leaving the Thymus. Thus disorders in the intestine can and do have a major influence on the Immune System and vice versa. Consult the medical texts for detailed explanations. The critical role of the bone marrow is explained as well as the functionality of the Thymus. The concert of action of these is also explained.

The texts on the causes of Crohn's disease are not decisive as to whether the disorder is a result or caused by the Immune System. There are also theories as to whether the cause is a virus or bacterium. There are many papers that associate **RA** with Crohn's disease. Usually the **RA** occurs after the Crohn's Disease (CD), but not always. Many times the patient does **NOT** have the genetic marker HLA- B27. It may be that a low level of Crohn's disease may be present , and undetected, and have a very important part in the development of **RA**. Almost **all** patients that had a bad small intestinal staple procedure for weight control contracted **RA**. Is there a strong causal connection ? Could effective treatment of CD prevent severe **RA** ? Is this being investigated ?

Older research seeks to connect Mycobacterium paratuberculosis with CD. Newer papers investigate genetics and viral causatives. There are many papers on the viral causative. Many papers address the role of viruses, and the loss of tolerance to self-antigens ; Many more papers point to the role of viral damage, and the breakdown of self tolerance. I think that the Researchers are getting close to the truth, and can explain the mechanisms quite well. Thus ,the link appears to be strong that viral damage will lead to Immune dysfunction; this viral attack may be accompanied by a bacterial action that makes the mechanism unclear. It appears that both are needed. Once the Immune System is uncoded on a molecular level and "thinks " on a molecular level that self is an antigen, then the autoimmune response is in full bloom and the disease may take form such as **RA** or MS or whatever. From the work to date, the leading contender appears to be HHV-6 in the viral domain or for **RA** possibly Morbillivirus (a mutant species), and some form of Streptococci (?) in the bacterial , plus, but not always some genetic marker such as HLA-B27 or HLA-DR4 (for **RA**). It also appears that a long undiagnosed problem in the gut (small intestine) may play a significant role especially for **RA**. The exact species of pathogen will also have a mimicry ability that will further confuse the Immune System. It is my belief that well directed research should reveal the exact pathogen and that this is in progress (I hope).

Meanwhile , aggressive therapy should assume that the above **may** be the true path and fully address the pathogens role, and the gut ,and the role of the Thymus. It may also be possible that some insects and people are acting as vectors for the disease. The most likely culprits are spouses or close friends or relatives and insects (unknown) . Experiments with large populations of mice should be done to properly identify relevant pathogens and combinations of pathogens and genetics. Effective therapies must be devised. Next ,experiments on primates and finally on humans. This may be in progress.

The current knowledge is expanding, but no cure is presently available, and the exact mechanism and treatment is under study and evolution. Doctors and patients must use an aggressive treatment for arthritis that begins to match the aggressive character of the disorder itself.

Anna's Story Continues..........

" If ever two were one, then surely we.
If ever man were loved by his wife, then thee:
If ever wife was happy in a man,
Compare with me, ye women , if you can.
I prize thy love more than the whole mines of gold
Or of all the riches that the East doth hold.
My love is such that rivers cannot quench,
Nor ought but love from thee, give recompense.
Thy love is such that I can no way repay,
The heavens reward thee manifold, I pray,
Then while we live, in love, let's so persevere
That when we live no more, we may live ever. "

To My Dear and Loving Husband by Anne Bradstreet (1612-1672)

Our wedding was in a small Chapel in the Kingdom by the Sea. The bride was in white as well as the groom. It was a happy wedding and a happy day. The Sun rolled back, and the sky was a blue such as never seen by man. The Seagulls circled in glee, and the Heavens sighed in Pleasure...... The Minister was very pleased and a new life had begun...... That of Anna and I. The Minister even went to the reception, and partook of the some of the refreshments. He was in good spirits; you might even say that he was effervescent.

" Behold you are beautiful, my love,
behold you are beautiful !
.....
You are fair ,my love:
there is no flaw in you

……..

How much better is your love

and the fragrance of your oils than any spice !

…………..

Let my beloved come to his garden ,

and eat its choicest fruits.

Excerpts from *The Song of Solomon* (King James Version-read it all-it is quite beautiful)

This time and events were marked by a ***special*** **Gold Cord in Anna's Bible**. She must have read this to her self at times- I never knew, until now. I knew that she loved the story of Ruth . She really loved me and I her; ours was a marriage truly conceived in Heaven by **God**. She must have been one of his Angels sent to me. I have never nor since met or experienced such profound Love. Most of us simply read of such- to experience such is to partake of Heaven itself. The utter Joy is almost impossible to describe.

There was an abundance of good times, and we had a life that many truly good marriages reflect. We had a very special relation to each other and this never changed with time or any event that transpired. Of all the changing venues and visitudes of life, this was constant.

" **Shall I compare thee to a summer's day** ?
Thou art more lovely and more temperate:
Rough winds do shake the darling buds of May,
And summer's lease hath all too short a date:
Sometimes too hot the eye of heaven shines,
And often is his gold complexion dimm'd :
And every fair from fair something declines,
By chance, or by nature changing course untrimm'd:
But thy eternal summer shall not fade,
Nor lose possession of that fair Thou ow'st,
Nor shall death brag Thou wanderst in his shade,
When in eternal lines to time Thou grow'st;
So long as men can breathe, or eyes can see,

So long lives this, and gives life to Thee."

Sonnet 18 by William Shakespeare (with some minor modifications)

‘

Some Thoughts

There is an experiment in particle physics that is very interesting and very intriguing. If you have an atom or molecule, and you separate the electrons from the orbital shells, you will find a very interesting behavior of electrons that previously shared a similar orbit about a common nucleus of neutrons and protons. It is called the paired particle experiment and is still a mystery. If you have these particles in remote areas from each other locations, you can perturb the orbit of one and its previous pair will experience a similar perturbation. Remember that these particles are now far removed from one another and no emf, no magnetic, no gravitational, etc. force can effect both if the separation is great in space. Yet if you do the experiment properly, the previously paired electron will experience exactly the same effect as the one that is perturbed by the experimenter. By all the known laws of physics, this should not happen, but it does. This may seem trivial but it is not. It is as if the very elemental particles that make up the universe have properties and characteristics that are very common. It is almost as if there was some innate properties in the most elemental of particles.

Now expand your horizon a bit. Consider the Universe. The vastness, the vast array of stars, the collections of stars, and the very scale. It is believed that the Universe is expanding and that it began about 15 billion years ago. If you turn on your TV late at night and tune it to a station that has stopped broadcasting, you can find direct evidence of this event. The static is strong and noisy. This is the background energy of the formation of the universe. The state of the residual energy is about 4 degrees Kelvin in a broadband mode. Your TV ,if used with a simple antenna , can detect this energy since the device is made to detect and amplify signals in the low microvolt range and at frequencies of 50 Mega Hertz and above . This is same energy content as the formational energy. This was measured much more accurately, and with more precision and information with the COBE (Cosmic Background Explorer) satellite. Thus, some process or **Something** that pervades, and is a part of all matter had something in common with or was apart or a cause of this event or all of the above. We are a very unique species in that we can recognize such, and recognize our own being and relate this being to others and to the Cosmos. I am certain that other species can do this, but they lack the language and cognitive skills that we do. This is both good and perhaps not so good; and it has its down side. We know and experience the marvel of Creation , but we also experience pain and suffering and the apparent demise of that which is good. Of course in doing so we must account for our very finite abilities and ability to understand.

Life

It is thought by some that life is a very unique and unusual phenomena. This is true that it is unique and unusual, but there is more. The very nature of beings, from the smallest microbe such as a virus to the very largest mammal or the mammal with the greatest intelligence and awareness, is similar. If you consider DNA itself and examine the complex protein structure, you find a high -almost phenomenal level of intelligence in the coding. There is something here that pervades, that comprises our very being. This is us; this is something more than we completely understand. For instance, how is that some beings reproduce and simply produce a copy of the original subject to mutations. Other seek to enrich the genetic code and produce something new . Still others can actually decide on the mode of reproduction (very primitive (?) creatures). We live in a sea of life. Some forms rely on others for survival; some forms convert energy from the Sun directly; some forms depend on these life forms for survival; and some forms depend on the latter for survival.. There are some very unique forms that can make choices, and are aware of their own existence and mortality. We are a highly evolved species. We have cognitive powers that are astounding. And we are still changing. The process never stops. We recognize and we feel. We feel strongly for one another; we feel that we do not completely or even partly understand.

We are indeed fortunate and unfortunate. We can chose; we can do good; conversely we can do the opposite. Our being is much greater than any part, and we have a persistent continuity. We are probably not unique in the Universe. The very nature of matter dictates that there are similar beings in the Universe. There may also be dissimilar beings that are equally intelligent and perhaps even more intelligent. The problem we have is that many species such as microbes live in us, and use us for their survival. Some are benign; some actually help us daily. Unfortunately, some species in their quest for survival do us immense harm. That is where the Immune System lives and works. It deals daily with these species on a molecular level. If the wrong molecular signal is given to the receptors of the Immune System, the being is perceived to be alien and posses alien qualities; then, the Immune System responded to this signal as what is called a response to an antigen. Thus to preserve Self, and the being that is us; the Immune System must attack and eliminate the foreign matter or beings. This then is a part of our being. The receptors in parts of the Immune System that respond to these alien molecular signatures can respond and recognize around one billion signatures (this number seems to grow as the texts become more modern and the understanding grows). We even have a system of cells assigned to carry and store information. Thus , when we have been attacked, and the attack was repelled, the information needed to repel a new attack is quickly retrieved and used. The medical term is Immunity. The Immune System in correct function is possessed of a beauty and coherence and intelligence that is truly inspiring.

The problem is that some organisms may have learned tricks to foil this response, and the response by the Immune System is inappropriate. Thus, the disorders related to the Immune System occur. Thus, it is not a simple or easy task to discern why the Immune response seems to be inappropriate. The problem is innate. The microbes have some intelligence and will mutate and also try to disguise their identity. Such is their nature. Our nature is to fight and thwart this attempt to diminish our being. We understand suffering in ourselves and others and strive to eliminate such. **This is our nature; this our Destiny: To care for one another-Nothing in Life is greater. To work for each other is an expression of our higher Being. It is something we Must do**. We actually do this every day, it is not always apparent. Doctors do this every day. They understand the nature of the battle and the conflict between us and the sea of microbes that would like to live at our expense. It is a battle that can be helped with the proper medications and treatments. The science of medicine is evolving just as surely as we are.

Chapter 14

RAX AND COMPANIONS

Anna's Story Continues....

Today was difficult. I could feel the slow movement and the rapid progression of life around me as if in some juxtaposition of unknown meaning and depth . Today was exactly one year to the day since Anna departed. The time was about 11:40 A.M., June 12, 1997. I was called to come to the hospital-there was a conveyance in the message that it was urgent that I come-I did. Never have I felt such pain and sorrow intermingled and with such intensity in all my life. Anna was lifeless and quite cool. As I gazed on her countenance I knew that that was not Anna- She had left and this was apparently what was left of her temporal residence on this planet known as earth. My expressions of grief must have and were quite loud as if my plaintive cries could influence the events preceding-No ,No, not so . I can still feel and picture this event a year later. I know precisely what was said and what was done. The very being that made my being worth being had ceased to exist ; the grief and feelings overwhelmed completely. All of the pain and sorrow and misadventure of mankind seemed to descend on my being. My very Soul wailed to God and his Angels. I knew that indeed I had talked with an Angel of God and the very simple dialogue was eloquent , " **She has suffered enough .**" This helped assuage my grief in the true knowledge that God had called her home and that further suffering was pointless-I must accept this and I do. I feel very privileged to be so honored by the very Creator of us and his infinite Love for us is always there and expressed. I know that this event was for the best, but of course still difficult. All around me were very supportive and this was greatly appreciated. Man can be Noble when he tries-it is part of our nature. We should do, act, and be such with more frequency. We are all God's children and we need to interact and help each other as much as possible. This is our intrinsic nature.

About sometime after lunch I was ahead in my work and decided to search for news of any progress in Medicine and in particular-Immunology and Rheumatology. I visited some of the usual sites and was about to stop when there before disbelieving eyes was **RAX.** Science will now prevail and I shall explain this in their profound vernacular.

RAX and COMPARIOTS

" Good ideas are not adopted automatically. They must be driven into practice with courageous impatience. "

Admiral Hyman G. Rickover

The work was dome by Dr. Joel B. Baseman and Dr. Joseph G. Tully of the University of Texas Health Science Center at San Antonio. The was supported by the University of Texas and the National Institute of Health. This may obtained from *Emerging Infectious Diseases*, 3(1):21-32, 1997, Centers for Disease Control. The information and some text may also be obtained from NIH or the University of Texas or Medline. Go to any library if you have trouble and they will provide one copy for a nominal charge (about 15c per page). The keyword for a search is mycoplasma and arthritis on the Internet. Additional sources will be referenced and also noted fully as to who and where. Of course, the vernacular is weighty and I shall attempt to make it understandable. If you have a medical background, the original sources are to be consulted. The title of the article (there is a great profusion of these) is: Mycoplasmas: Sophisticated, Reemerging, and Burdened by Their Notoriety . There are 79 references for this article alone-Impressive. There many other articles but this is truly the Pioneer, the Great Explanation.

I have early referenced these beings (Mycoplasmas) but as many before me have dismissed the work as not Proven-a Big Mistake. Science should not be subject to prejudice and must be examined in a truly objective manner. The authors explain this with a quote by Thomas Huxley. You must read this full article to fully appreciate what is said . A mycoplasma is one of the smallest self replicating beings alive , and is a bacteria, but is very small at about 0.3 microns. Something this small can be seen only with an Electron Microscope. This bacteria has no cell wall. It has a very compact genetic structure. It also has and requires cholesterol for function such as plants. It can pass through so called bacterial filters with no problem. There can be as many as a billion in a ml and no turbidity (clear) can not be discerned by normal tests. In addition, there is no change in pH level . All usual tests will not detect their presence and outside the body or in vitro as opposed to in vivo, they quickly disappear as if phantoms. These fellows are very particular, and require just the right temperature and saline content as well as other necessary environmental factors. For the most part when you attempt to separate them from their host cells, they disappear. Thus, many researches declare with *profound* authority that they do not exist. They do- and these guys are parasites. They have little tips and enter into the cells of their host or are very closely attached to the surface. When observation is attempted, if great care is not observed, they appear to be part of the host cell. If done correctly, they can be seen with the Electron microscope as attached to the host with their little tips called organelles. Many also assume they are an intrinsic part of the benign flora and fauna that exist in our systems. Not so ! Some species will be explained, and are killers. They do not kill the cell per se (sometimes) but induce an immune response that kills the host. The Army of the Immune is activated and attacks but ends by attacking Self since these parasites are part of self. This mechanism is complex ,and the reader is strongly advised to read the Journal and articles by the experts. These fellows are some our worst enemies , but are rarely treated as such. This truly amazes me. If you read these articles they have some excellent pictures of these bacteria and their action on the cell. It is obvious that no good is intended and they live at your expense and degraded health-perhaps worse. The author says that they are " true card carrying pathogens " . Aptly said.

It is shown that some of these organisms are responsible for :

1. **Pneumonia**-so called "walking pneumonia "
2. AIDS complications
3. **Heart** disease
4. GI diseases such as **Chron's Disease**
5. A **Host** of auto immune disease such as the various arthritic disorders
6. Great suspicion as to be the **cause of Tumors** and tumor growth
7. **Septicemia** infections in the initial stage
8. Chronic fatigue

Many other disorders

There are about 200 known species which probably means that there are at least 100 times this in existence. These bacteria may be responsible for untold human, and animal misery and death. We have recognized the enemy. The attack must begin- continued suffering is totally unacceptable. Those that have ears must listen; those that have eyes shall see. Scientific analysis and discovery will proceed ; indifference and disbelief will have to be corrected.

One of the mycoplasma suspected in the arthritic diseases is called *M .genitalium.* That for pneumonia is called *M. pneumonia.* In the joint tissue, we find *M. hominus.* **Fatal septicemia** is associated with *M. arginni.* There are many, many more, but for the investigation of **RA** these species and some others will be proposed to explain some of the causative mysteries of some diseases .

Some early research connected Mycobacterium paratuberculosis with Chron's disease (CD). The two mycoplasma recent reveled to have a major effect in both are *M. pneumonia* and *M .genitalium.* It has also been noted that severe **RA is almost always concurrent with CD.** Anna had both and the literature abounds with the same information ,but no is sure of the connection. Dr. Baseman and Dr. Tully have made a remarkable revelation.

An article by B.C. Cole and M.M. Griffiths in *Arthritis and Rheumatology,* Volume 36, Issue , pp. 994-1002 explains a class of mycoplasma arthritis superantigen may induce the activation of self reactive T cells. To test this theory, the authors created a superantigen from a natural variant of murine arthitogenic mycoplasma ; they called the variant MAM. This mycoplasma was found to induce and/or trigger **RA** in mice with a remarkable cause and effect relationship. The authors conclude that it is indeed possible that similar superantigens may induce or play a significant role in **RA.**

T. Schaeverbeke and co-authors in *The Journal of Clinical Pathology*, Vol. 49, Issue 10, pp. 824-828 found that the mycoplasma *M. fermentans* was present in the joints of a significant percentage of patients with inflammatory rheumatic disorders including RA. The method used is explained in the text. Previous attempts have not been successful since the technology need for the detection is somewhat new.

In Japan, H. Kaneoka and S. Naito in the journal, *Nippon Rinsho,* Vol. 55, Issue 6 , pp. 1363-1369 have also postulated the existence of similar superantigens as being responsible for a wide array of autoimmune diseases including RA . They refer to mycoplasma arthritis T cell mitogen as being arithogenic to mice. It is possible that the same is true in humans but work is not complete.

In Britain, B. Bannwarth ,C. Be′be′ar, and J. Dehais in *The British journal of Rheumatology* , Vol. 36, Issue 3, pp. 310-314 have detected mycoplasma by PCR procedures in over 200 synovial fluid samples. The mycoplasma were *hominus, fermentans,* and lessor percentages of *salivarium, orale,* and some *Ureaplasma urealyticum.*

When searching for correlation's, the number of articles has risen dramatically in the last year. The number of correlation's has increased from 10-100 to at least 24,000 on one try. To me, this is of some significance. It does not prove the postulate that mycoplasmas are the cause of auto immune disorders, but it does suggest strongly that many consider their causative effect very seriously. The number of articles and authors is so extensive that reader is advised to consult Medline for a listing. Thus, it appears that there is much credence to this hypothesis that mycoplasma are involved in the inception of RA and many other autoimmune disorders.

Dr. Baseman and Dr. Tully note that the mycoplasmas have a homology to mammalian structural protein ; this property lends to molecular mimicry. The doctors are saying that the embedded mycoplasma is so close in protein structure to the host that the they have the quality of mimicry. The immune system is not fooled but since the structure is so close to that of self cells, the antibodies produced also attack self cells as well as the mycoplasmas. The description in the article is much more complex and should be consulted. These fellows do some bad things to the cells (*Shame !*) . Dr. Baseman says they: (caution-my version of what was written-to try to keep this remotely understandable for those with no medical training)

1. Generate hydrogen peroxide- cause cell damage
2. Compete for cell nutrients-cells die or are damaged
3. Create surface layers such that immune attack is thwarted
4. This is so unusual that the author must be quoted directly , " high -frequency phase and antigenic variation, which results in surface diversity and possible avoidance of protective host immune defenses."
5. Secrete some really bad enzymes which disrupt the tissue and result in disorganization, and chromosomal aberrations (not nice fellows !) .
6. They have the ability to hide in your cells in a latent or chronic state and are resistant to both immune attack and drug therapies.

Of all the disorders that Dr. Baseman examines, the logic and evidence for causal effects in AIDS, Chron's Disease, and RA and other arthritides is most convincing. The antigen in CD is *M . pneumonia.* The very treatments used may, " precipitate the onset of acute exacerbation's of chronic inflammatory bowel disease." This is most distressing.

The RA has the observed occurrence of Mycoplasma and Ureaplasma. Some of the specie have been previously described and observed. It is suggested that a suitable antibiotic be developed. The current antibiotics such as tetracycline, etc. may be used but require long term administration to have any effect. Thus, a potential solution to the mystery of the cause of RA has been grandly elucidated.

Now, if we reexamine Anna's history, we find :

1. She had pneumonia
2. Her mother died of cancer, possible gene defect or marker as previously explained
3. She was female and over 40 when the disease started
4. She had Chron's disease but not until later

If just one case is cited, the evidence is not conclusive for the all cases. There have been many studies and most of these do suspect mycoplasma. The exact species is not conclusive. In addition, there are three types of RA . Type I responds to almost any treatment-hence the quackery associated with many so called cures. Type II responds to most of the medications with real relief for the patient. Type III responds only to very aggressive treatment. Even if treated (as done currently), Type III is fatal. The treatment and the disease result in a progression of effects. Thus, mycoplasma is probably one of the causative agents especially for Type I and II. Type III may have additional specie of mycoplasma and possibly virus such as Epstein-Barr. In Type III , the immune response is such to cause great damage to the host (Self). Thus treatment such as prolonged use of tetracycline would probably be of some value, but, it may not " cure " Type III. Nevertheless, for the more benign types, some antibiotic ,especially, on such as tetracycline is clearly indicated. Compared to the other medications, tetracycline can do little harm unless there a pronounced allergy. It is one of the few antibiotics that can be give for a prolonged period without serious problems with other pathogens. Thus, as a "blanket ", until the exact cause is known, the prolonged use of tetracycline is advised.

There is a very new medicine that can effectively control and effectively treat Chron's disease. His medicine is called ISIS 2302 and was described in the June 1998 issue of *Gastroenterology*. The drug is made by Isis Pharmaceuticals and is in Phase II trials. The compound is an antisense inhibitor of a intercellular adhesion molecule that is known in a to exist in inflammatory conditions. The molecular cluster is known as CD-54. This new drug suppresses and inhibits the formation of CD-54. The results of the studies are explained in the Journal by Dr. Bruce Yacyshyn of the University of Alberta. The drug is so effective that between 33 and 50% of the patient population were able to reduce or eliminate all current medications. All open fistula healed and an many were free of any obstructive indications. The restoration of normal bowel mucosal integrity was impressive. The exact nature of the drug is explained to some extent in the article in *Gastroenterology*.

The curious nature of Methotrexate needs to be reexamined. Why is it so effective ? The compound is a potent inhibitor of the conversion of folic acid to its usable form as a tetrahydrofolate. This compound is used for DNA synthesis. Thus, Methotrexate is a very potent inhibitor of DNA synthesis which accounts for its toxicity. In very low dosages, it can be used and most can tolerate low doses over effective treatment periods. It was first used for cancer. The next use was for psoriatic conditions. It was noticed that the patients with arthritis, especially active, aggressive forms such as RA responded well and achieved partial remissions. The use of Methotrexate is so effective that it has extended applications to many other disorders.

The key to the mystery is the compound is a potent inhibitor of the conversion of folic acid to the folate (tetrahydrofolate). This actually an enzyme with a long name and is abbreviated as DHFR and Methotrexate is called MTX. You may ask why this is so exciting and with good reason. Why is the drug so effective ? An answer is suggested by consulting a text on the development of drugs to combat and kill pathogens and the strategy used or such efforts. There are many texts and publications, but the one I have is *Emerging Targets in Antibacterial and Antifungal Chemotherapy* Edited by Joyce Sutcliffe and Nafsika H. Georgopapadakou and is published by Chapman and Hall . If Chapter 22 is consulted, the information combined with the current information is riveting, to say the least. Chapter 22 is by Gregg Y. Lipschik and Joseph A. Kovacs and is titled : *Chemotherapeutic Targets in Pneumocystis carnii.* Pages 570-577 are ultra important. Here , the folate metabolism of the microbe is described in detail. Guess what- these bacteria need and have a folate mechanism and do produce DHFR . Here it is explained that MTX is a potent DHFR inhibitor but the MTX requires a folate specific carrier (the drug must be lipid soluble to cross the cell membrane). This is usually not found in microbes. However a close relative of MTX called Trimetrexate which an analog of MTX can cross the cell membrane wall and provide disruption of DHFR. This is called TMTX. TMTX is very, very toxic since it is toxic to the host as well as the pathogen microbe. This toxicity can be controlled very simply by the concurrent administration of calcium leucovorin.

Now what microbe does not have a cell wall per se and is even in its name- *Mycoplasma* !!!!!!!!! Thus, Golden Boy can interfere and severely disrupt folate metabolism and DNA synthesis in *Mycoplasma*. Now, it is clear why it works. It does much more than suppress DNA synthesis of the host, it, MTX can attack that of a microbe without a cell wall. TMTX can disrupt a bacteria with a cell wall. This conclusion is not in any literature and it may be in error, but the logic may be correct. MTX is effective against the Immune response and in addition attacks one (there may be more) of the causes of RA. Thus, the mechanism of MTX is to attack the folate formation of the bacterium without a cell wall (dead buggies !!!) as well as suppress the Immune response by DNA suppression. Thus MTX or Methotrexate is the drug of choice for RA. To be certain of success, it may interesting to co-administer

MTX and TMTX with calcium leucovorin to mice first and then higher mammals and finally humans. This may provide a true cure. The combination of MTX and TMTX with calcium leucovorin and other therapies may be the solution . The other therapies such as those of the Naval Research Institute are also front contenders since they have no toxicity problems and do make the Immune as Nature intended. However, the reeducation of the Immune system does not attack the pathogen which may be the root cause of the disease(s). Thus both are needed : MTX and the NRI approach should be thoroughly tested. This was pioneered by Dr. David Harlan and Dr. Allan Kirk and many other Naval Research Institute Researchers as well as Researchers from the University of Wisconsin, and Scientists from Biogen and Genetics Institute of Cambridge .

Golden Boy and Immune Reeducation are almost certain to offer real relief and perhaps a cure. The true RAX may be a combination of a specie or many Mycoplasma as well as a virus. The way is clear-it just needs to be done.

A very interesting first chapter in the same book, *Emerging Targets in Antibacterial and Antifungal Chemotherapy* is by Akira Imada and Kunimoto Hotta entitled : Historical Perspectives of Approaches to Antibiotics Discovery. Page 8 is of interest for RA causes and possible treatment. Here the action of the fluoroquinolones is reported. Of even greater interest is the information about the inhibitors of folate metabolism in bacteria. This research lead to the discovery of diazaquinomycins A and B and AM-8042. This work is further elaborated in papers by S.M. Omura, et. Al. : Screening for new antifolates of microbial origin and a new antifolate, AM-8402. *Journal of Antibiotics* ,38 ,1016-1024, 1985 and more recently in 1996 by the same author, Omura, in Philosophy of New Drug Discovery in *Microbiology Review* : pp. 259-279. This class of drugs may be a good choice to use against Mycoplasma since it acts very strongly as does Methotrexate and to a lesser extent, tetracycline to disrupt DNA synthesis in certain bacteria . It is possible that these drugs in combination or used in a defined selective process would offer some real hope for the cure of RA. In addition, there is some work on a compound related to diazaquinomycins called 3-floro-1-aza- and 1,8- diazaanthaquinones that have the ability to inhibit the growth of various tumors. The work was done by Dr. M. T. Ramos, et. Al of the Universidad Complutense of Madrid , Spain. It is reported in English in *Farmaco*, 51 (5) : pp. 375-379, May, 1996. One of the links that always seem to appear is the link between compounds used for cancer and autoimmune treatments and currently-AIDS treatments. I currently do not know what is the link but hope to have some insight soon.

Thus, currently effective therapies emerge that can be used today :

1. Identify the severity of the RA ; If class I or II almost all the traditional therapies will work
2. If Severe Class III exists, then all the conventional treatments should not be tried. Why use medications that are known not to work for a patient for any time at all. After millions of cases, this should be clear. Thus, if you consult the literature, you find that indeed that this what many leading Research Centers, Books, and Journals strongly advocate for patients with severe RA. Consult any on-line source or book. Consult *Drug and Therapeutical Perspectives* , 1998 by Adis International Limited, etc., etc.. Consult *Clinician Reviews* , 1996 ff. . Use aggressive therapy against an aggressive disease while the patient is in fairly good condition. Do not wait until severe progression to use some of these really effective but somewhat toxic agents. The use of Methotrexate as early as possible should be done.
3. Treat the anemia with Anadrol
4. Use COX-2 for pain or NSAIDs that can be tolerated
5. Prescribe Tetracycline for at least 6 months just as the disease is first noted
6. Try Enbrel by Immunex
7. Try Zenapax ®

The physician must be a strong advocate of early aggressive and effective treatment. Reverse the pyramid treatment regime-it doesn't work for Class III RA . The treatment of RA is changing …The patient must benefit from this work.

" To go against the dominant thinking of your friends, of most of the people you see every day, is perhaps the most difficult act of heroism you can perform. "

Theodore H. White

For the physician, this advice may not be well received ,since it contradicts much of what is taught and practiced. I am well aware of the difficulty, but the patient is the first priority and not the opinion of peers. Of all that can be done, restoration of health and life is the most important task. Money, opinions, convention, standard practice and any other consideration pales compared to that of true help to the sufferer. No sacrifice or effort is too great to accomplish this mission. It is easy for me to say and write this, but I did my best to help and now feel that I must help others, regardless. It may be that many of the suggestions and information is flawed but there is some new insight and direction that will give hope to the hopeless and relief for the patient with severe RA.

" Love has no desire but to fulfill itself. To melt and be like a running brook that sings its melody to the night. To wake at dawn with a winged heart and give thanks for another day of Loving. "

Kahlil Gibran

" For as Much as you do for the least of these, you do for Me. "

Jesus

Anna's Story Continues ....

I was typing away and looked up the other night and something very strange occurred. A large bright beam of light seemed to emerge from the wall to my left. There was no light there. In addition, another small beam light brightly emanated from my wedding ring and reached to the full extent of the room both left and right of the ring. At first I was somewhat alarmed and later curious. What is this ? I had noticed that there was some fog outside. I also noted that the phenomena stopped when I removed my glasses. I surmised that the glasses had a slight smattering of oil from my skin and that was causing, with the very high humidity, the appearance of the beam of light as a result of some polarity effect combined with condensation that made the beam of light from the light on my left rotate about 90 degrees and appear to emanate from the wall. Satisfied with this explanation, I continued to work (strange lights and all). Tonight, I did not clean the glasses and tried to repeat the observation- nothing ! No matter what I have tried, there is no light from the wall and none from the ring. I am indeed puzzled. Maybe it isn't humid enough. Actually, it is more humid than last night . The light last night appeared about 10 P.M. It is now 8:30 , maybe again at 10, maybe not. I feel that I can discern the cause of this but so far am mystified. I feel that whatever it is, it is possible that it will reoccur . I also noticed that my left hand seemed to glow- I haven't the slightest explanation for that.

Doctors and Nurses in the Kingdom by the Sea

Anna had many doctors and nurses. They were all good to her and made a distinct impression on me. They were very professional but at the same time very personable and conveyed a sense that they were truly trying to help. Anna looked forward to her visits with her family physician ; they had the greatest chats and she usually got somewhat better. Her doctor was her friend, and in an emergency, she gave me her home telephone number. I used it only in true emergencies since I perceived that she (Anna's Family Doctor) had very little free time and I did not want to disturb her unless absolutely necessary. She was very frustrated by the lack of effective medications for **RA** . Her office manager and Anna were great friend and had very animated conversations. When Anna would call, the office manager would ask, " Are you a strawberry or a rudabaker today ? " If a strawberry, she was in good spirits and feeling better; if a rudabaker, she was not well.

She had two orthopedic surgeons and both were very helpful. They performed miracles and restored the use of her hands, feet, and one hip. They and their staff were friendly and always willing to discuss the illness and what could be done. In addition, Anna had tow full surgeons of a caliber approaching nobility in their abilities and manner. I was very impressed by these fellows. Both were directly responsible for saving her life, more than once. If we had any problems, they allowed me to call their beeper wherever they were. Doctors are like this in the Magic Kingdom by the Sea.

Anna also had a gastroentroentologist and a heart specialist. Both did good work. I was really impressed with the work done at the hospital by the heart specialist. He essentially restored not only her heart but her vascular system improved and her ulcers and vasculitis disappeared. In about 3 days, she almost looked normal and was very pink and healthy looking. He ,also, was always available for consultation.

The nurses were Anna's friends and continuously helped. I stayed at various hospitals and they would teach me wound care and techniques for the care of the very distressed. This was very helpful. I also learned much from her home care nurses-they also were good . On each visit, I was given a lesson on various techniques. I was the 24 hour nurse. People were like this and Anna instantly made friends with all she came in contact with. I was always impressed by how she impressed others and made them feel good when she in such pain.

We tried mightily to make her well. At one time, I thought we were succeeding ,but there always seemed to be complications. Anna had many friends and was loved and liked by all. In spite of all the difficulties, we had a good life together. Her life was a tribute to courage and love as she personified both. Just to meet and talk to her would make you happy. The doctors and nurses sensed this and tried every known principle of medicine and science. We all tried ,and tried with a passion.

The Sun shone brightly in the Kingdom by the Sea , but then one day a chill wind took my Anna Lee...

Chapter 15
Ending

" **Our revels now are ended**. These are our actors,
As I foretold you, were all spirits, and
Are melted into air, into thin air;
And, like the baseless fabric of this vision,
The cloud-capped towers, the gorgeous places,
The solemn temples, the great globe itself,
Yea, all which it inherit shall dissolve,
And like, like his insubstantial pageant faded,
Leave not a rack behind. ***We are such stuff***
As dreams are made on, and our little life
Is rounded with a sleep. *"*

(William Shakespeare-*Our Revels Now Are Ended*)

Prologue

Anna brought light into my life and many others. Just to be in her presence was to experience this feeling of brightness and happiness. Confucius said " He (or she) who wished to secure the good of others has already secured his (or her) own. " This was true of Anna. Her life was devoted to others and made many people happy in ways that could not be explained.

We had a very special relationship and this will exist forever. Even the cat, Tut ,was part of the relationship. Somehow he knew and felt our special little universe. I never had to correct him after he was trained and an adult cat. He even had nicknames that he also understood to be his. His sickness and demise immediately preceded Anna's.

"How true, dear, my love is;
Too great to compare,
Truer than the stars,
That shoot from their sphere ;
....

Even time must change

    To eternity.

Oh ! there is no changing in my love for thee.

………………………………….

Fear not that pale death

Will drift us apart:

Ah ! death cannot sever

The love in my heart.

When we reach heaven

We shall find our own ;

I'm told we will know there

As we are known."

James E, McGirt (James Ephraim) , *True Love* in *For Your Sweet Sake, Poems,* 1906 (Highly abridged and modified)

The **Angel of Death** spoke to me very few words but I am very privileged to have this message. The message was very short, " **Richard ! She has suffered enough .** " Thus, God himself brought Anna back to his Being. This is hard to comprehend and is stated as fact since this did occur.

I am aware that there are many that will say that this was simply the imagination of a grieved spouse. This not so ! I am a scientist and very much so. I even doubted this at first, but the event was so compelling that I cannot erase it. I am changed. I can feel other's love and suffering ; I feel great privilege for this and thank God for his Love . Anna is not here ; she is with God and I feel this, strongly.

Anna

(In Memorial, June 12, 1998)

Anna brought Light into my life and to many others. Just to be in Her presence was to experience this feeling of ***brightness and happiness***.

" He who wished to secure the Good of others has already secured his own. " (*Confucius*) This was true of Anna. Her life was devoted to others, and she made many people happy in ways that could not be explained.

My Love for you will shine as the Sun with the Depth of the Universe. When you see a baby smile, or see the Sun or Stars in God's Universe, you will feel this Eternal Love. At eve, the gentle breeze will whisper this Message of Love and Caring to the very Heart of your Being.

This is Our Eternal Love.

" Then while we live, in love, let's so persevere

That when we live no more, we may live ever. "

To My Dear and Loving Husband by Anne Bradstreet (1612-1672)

Until, we meet again

Richard L.

Anna (In Memoriam , June 12, 1999)

Anna lived with no other thought than to Love and to be loved by me. Her being was my Universe , and just to be near her made me happy. Our Love was constant ,and the very Sun looked to it for Light. So, my Love will shine for Anna as the Sun with the Depth of the Universe. When you see the Sun or Stars in God's Universe, you will feel this Eternal Love. At eve, the gentle breeze will whisper this Message of Love and Caring to the very Heart of your Being. Time will never diminish my thoughts and Love. A part of you still lives in me ,and will forever ; this will be so forever until Ever becomes Never and we are part of God.

Your Loving Husband
Richard

REFERENCES*

(Background Only)

*** References used in text are quoted as used therein**

1. Firestein G.S.; Echeverri F; Yeo M; Zvaifler NJ; Green DR: Somatic mutations in the p53 tumor suppressor gene in rheumatoid arthritis synovium, *Proceedings of the National Academy of Science*, U S A, 1997 Sep 30;94(20):10895-10900

2. Firestein G.S.; Nguyen K; Aupperle K.R.; Yeo M.; Boyle D.L.; Zvaifler NJ : Apoptosis in rheumatoid arthritis p53 overexpression in rheumatoid arthritis synovium, *American Journal of Pathology* ,1996 Dec;149(6):2143-2151

3. Segal, Benjamin M.;. Klinman ,Dennis M; and Shevach, Ethan M.: Microbial Products Induce Autoimmune Disease by an IL-12-Dependent Pathway, *The Journal of Immunology* Vol. 158, No. 11 Issue of 06-01-97 pp. 5087 - 5090

4. Offers E, Herbort C, Dumke K, Schneider H, Kolloch : Complicated course of rheumatoid arthritis with pulmonary involvement, myocardial fibrosis and sleep apnea syndrome ,*R Pneumologie* 1996 Dec;50(12):906-911

5. Schiff M : Emerging treatments for rheumatoid arthritis ,*American Journal of Medicine*,1997 Jan 27;102(1A):11S-15S

6. Conaghan PG, Lehmann T, Brooks P : Disease-modifying antirheumatic drugs, *Current Opinion in Rheumatology*, 1997 May;9(3):183-190

7. Ferraccioli GF, Bambara LM, Ferraris M, Perpignano G, Cattaneo R, Porzio F, Accardo S, Mattara L, Zoppini A, Benucci M, Ostuni PA, Pasero G: Effects of cyclosporine on joint damage in rheumatoid arthritis, *The Italian Rheumatologists Study Group on Rheumatoid Arthritis*, 1997 May;15 Supplement 17:S83-S89

8. Phillips PE: Viral arthritis, *Current Opinion in Rheumatology*, 1997 Jul;9(4):337-344

9. Paul C, Le Tourneau A, Cayuela JM, Devidas A, Robert C, Molinie V, Dubertret L: Epstein-Barr virus-associated lymphoproliferative disease during Methotrexate therapy for psoriasis , *Archives of Dermatology* ,1997 Jul;133(7):867-871

10. Biasi D, Caramaschi P, Carletto A, Pacor ML, Bambara LM: The mechanisms of action of disease-modifying antirheumatic drugs: a review with emphasis on macrophage signal transduction and the induction of proinflammatory cytokines, *General Pharmacology*, 1997 Aug;29(2):127-150

11. Firestein, Gary S. MD; and Zvaifler, Nathan J. MD : Anticytokine Therapy in Rheumatoid Arthritis, *The New England Journal of Medicine,* Volume 337, Number 3, July 17, 1997

12. Mosebach S; Tromm A ; Wittenborg A; and May B: Rheumatoid disorders in Crohn disease and Ulcerative colitis, *Leber Magen Darm,* 25(2): 76-85 1995 Mar. Abteilumg f'lur Gastroenterologie, UnivesitI'astklinik Bochum

13. Horowitz, Edward A., MD; Lien, Elizabeth A., MD; Mycobacteria and Crohn's Disease, *Infect. Medicine,* 14(7): 569-573, 1997

14. Beauvais, C.; Le Quintrec, JL: Prier, A: Flipo RM ; Kahn MF; and Kaplan G: Destructive arthritis of the hip in Crohn disease, *Presse Med,* 24(33): 1555-8 1995 Nov.4, Service de Rheumatolgie, Hospital Saint -Antoine, Paris, France

15. Scarpa, R; Lubrano E; Castiglone F; Ames PR; and Oriente P : Juvenile rheumatoid Arthritis, Chron's disease and Turners syndrome: a novel association, *Clinical experimental Rheumatology,* 14(4): 449-50 1996 July-August

16. Holzman, David: When Defenders Turn Destroyers, *Insight,* February 29, 1988

17. Schmitz JL, Schell RF, Callister SM, Lovrich SD, Day SP, Coe JE: IgG2 and Lyme ,*Infectious Immunology* ,1992 Jul;60(7):2677-2682 ,Wisconsin State Laboratory of Hygiene, University of Wisconsin-Madison, 53706

18. Ralph C. Schimmer, Denis J. Schrier, Craig M. Flory, James Dykens, David K.-L. Tung, Peer B., Jacobson, Hans P. Friedl, Mary Carol Conroy, Beatrice Beck Schimmer, and Peter A. Ward Title: Streptococcal Cell Wall-Induced Arthritis, *The Journal of Immunology* ,Volume: 159 Number: 8 Pages: 4103-4108 10-15-97

19. Leo A. B. Joosten, Erik Lubberts, Monique M. A. Helsen, and Wim B. van den Berg : Dual Role of IL-12 in Early and Late Stages of Murine Collagen Type II Arthritis, *The Journal of Immunology* Volume: 159 Number: 8 Pages: 4094-4102 10-15-97

20. Gregorio Aversa, Benjamin G. Cocks, Reijo Luukkainen, Riitta Saario, Paavo Toivanen: Increased Expression of Signaling Lymphocytic Activation Molecule in Patients with Rheumatoid Arthritis and Its Role in the Regulation of Cytokine Production in Rheumatoid Synovium ,*The Journal of Immunology* ,Volume: 159 Number: 6 Pages: 2986-2993 09-15-97

21. Sanui, H., T. M. Redmond, S. Kotake, B. Wiggert, T. Tanaka, G. J. Chader, and I. Gery. 1990: Thymic Expression of Autoantigens Correlates with Resistance to Autoimmune Disease , *Current Eye Research*, 9:193, Laboratory of Immunology, National Eye Institute, National Institutes of Health, Bethesda, MD 20892 Howard Hughes Medical Institute-National Institutes of Health Research Scholars

22. Eguagu, Charled E., Charukammoetkanok, and Gery : Thymic Expression of Autoantigens Correlates with resistance to AutoImmune Disease, *The Journal of Immunology,* Vol. 159, No. 7 Issue of 10-01 pp. 3109-3112

23. Allan D. Kirk; David M. Harlan; Nicholas N. Armstrong; Thomas A. Davis; Yinchen Dong; Gary S. Gray; Xuening Hong; David Thomas; John H. Fechner Jr.; and Stuart J. Knechtle : CTLA4-Ig and anti-CD40 ligand prevent renal allograft rejection in primates, *Proceedings of the. National Academy of Science ,USA*, Vol. 94, pp. 8789-8794, August 1997

24. Nilsson IM, Lee JC, Bremell T, Ryden C, Tarkowski A: The role of staphylococcal polysaccharide microcapsule expression in septicemia and septic arthritis., *Infectious Immunology,* 1997 Oct;65(10):4216-4221

25. Burt RK : BMT (Bone Marrow Transplant) for severe autoimmune diseases: an idea whose time has come., *Oncology* (Huntingt) 1997 Jul;11(7):1001-1014

26. Marmont, AM : Stem cell transplantation for severe autoimmune disorders, with special reference to rheumatic diseases, *Journal of Rheumatology Suppl* 1997 May;48:13-18

27. Hamilton JA, Biggs JC, Atkinson K, Brooks PM : Bone marrow transplantation in auto-immune disease. , *Baillieres Clinical Rheumatology*, 1995 Nov;9(4):673-687

28. Snowden JA, Atkinson K, Kearney P, Brooks P, Biggs JC : Allogeneic bone marrow transplantation from a donor with severe active rheumatoid arthritis not resulting in adoptive transfer of disease to recipient. *Bone Marrow Transplant*, 1997 Jul;20(1):71-73

29. Moreland LW, Baumgartner SW, Schiff MH, Tindall EA, Fleischmann RM, Weaver AL, Ettlinger RE, Cohen S, Koopman WJ, Mohler K, Widmer MB, Blosch CM : Treatment of rheumatoid arthritis with a recombinant human tumor necrosis factor receptor (p75)-Fc fusion protein., *New England Journal of Medicine*, 1997 Jul 17;337(3):141-147

30. Moreland LW, Margolies G, Heck LW Jr., Saway A, Blosch C, Hanna R, Koopman WJ : Recombinant soluble tumor necrosis factor receptor (p80) fusion protein: toxicity and dose finding trial in refractory rheumatoid arthritis. , *Journal of Rheumatology*, 1996 Nov;23(11):1849-1855

31. Moreland LW, Pratt PW, Mayes MD, Postlethwaite A, Weisman MH, Schnitzer T, Lightfoot R, Calabrese L, Zelinger DJ, Woody JN, et al : Double-blind, placebo-controlled multicenter trial using chimeric monoclonal anti-CD4 antibody, cM-T412, in rheumatoid arthritis patients receiving concomitant Methotrexate, *Arthritis and Rheumatology*, 1995 Nov;38(11):1581-1588

32. Adachi Y; Hinoda Y; Takahashi H; Nakagawa N; Sakamoto H; Itoh F; Endo T; Suzuki S; Imai K : Rheumatoid arthritis associated with ulcerative colitis., *Journal of Gastroenterology*, 31(4):590-5 1996 Aug., First Department of Internal Medicine, Sapporo Medical University School of Medicine, Japan

33. Mosebach S; Tromm A; Wittenborg A; May B: Rheumatoid disorders in Crohn disease and

ulcerative colitis. Dominance of non-inflammatory factors., *Leber Magen Darm*, 25(2):76, 79-85 1995 Mar, Abteilung f-ur Gastroenterologie, Universit-atsklinik Bochum

34. Toussirot E; Wendling D. : Crohn's disease associated with seropositive rheumatoid arthritis. *Clinical Experimental Rheumatology* , 15(3):307-11 1997 May-Jun

35. Nelson EA; Gibson B : The management of leg ulcers in a patient with ulcerative colitis. This case study details the treatment of a patient with pyoderma gangrenosum on the shins of both legs. *Journal of Wound Care*, 4(9):391-3 1995 Oct

36. Helenius P; Turunen U; Stenman S; Sepp- K; Leirisalo-Repo M : Relationship between intestinal inflammation and arthritis, *Duodecim*, 110(1):19-26 1994, HYKS:n II sis_tautien klinikka, Helsinki

37. Breedveld ,FC : Early rheumatoid arthritis. Future treatment, *Baillieres Clinical Rheumatology*, 11(1):83-96 1997 Feb., Department of Rheumatology, Leiden University Hospital, The Netherlands

38. Haqqi TM; Qu XM; Anthony D; Ma J; Sy MS : Immunization with T cell receptor V beta chain peptides deletes pathogenic T cells and prevents the induction of collagen-induced arthritis in mice., *Journal of Clinical Investigation*, 97(12):2849-58 1996 Jun 15

39. Kaandorp CJ; Van Schaardenburg D; Krijnen P; Habbema JD; van de Laar MA , Jan van Breemen : Risk factors for septic arthritis in patients with joint disease. A prospective study., *Arthritis and Rheumatolgy*, 38(12):1819-25 1995 Dec., Institute for Rheumatology and Rehabilitation, Amsterdam, The Netherlands

40. Waisman A; Ruiz PJ; Hirschberg DL; Gelman A; Oksenberg JR; Brocke S; Mor F; Cohen IR; Steinman L : Suppressive vaccination with DNA encoding a variable region gene of the T-cell receptor prevents autoimmune encephalomyelitis and activates Th2 immunity., *National Medicine*, 2(8):899-905 1996 Aug. Department of Immunology, Weizmann Institute of Science, Rehovot, Israel

41. Li SG, Quayle AJ, Shen Y, Kjeldsen-Kragh J, Oftung F, Gupta RS, Natvig JB, Forre OT : Mycobacterium and human heat shock protein-specific Cytotoxic T lymphocytes in rheumatoid synovial inflammation., *Arthritis and Rheumatology* 1992 Mar;35(3):270-281

42. Holzman, David: When Defenders Turn Destroyers, *Insight,* February 29, 1988

43. Scarpa, R; Lubrano E; Castiglone F; Ames PR; and Oriente P : Juvenile rheumatoid Arthritis, Chron's disease and Turners syndrome: a novel association, *Clinical experimental Rheumatology,* 14(4): 449-50 1996 July-August

44. Beauvais, C.; Le Quintrec, JL: Prier, A: Flipo RM ; Kahn MF; and Kaplan G: Destructive arthritis of the hip in Crohn disease, *Presse Med,* 24(33): 1555-8 1995 Nov.4, Service de Rheumatolgie, Hospital Saint -Antoine, Paris, France

45. Horowitz, Edward A., MD; Lien, Elizabeth A., MD; Mycobacteria and Crohn's Disease, *Infect. Medicine,* 14(7): 569-573, 1997

46. Mosebach S; Tromm A ; Wittenborg A; and May B: Rheumatoid disorders in Crohn disease and Ulcerative colitis, *Leber Magen Darm,* 25(2): 76-85 1995 Mar. Abteilumg f'lur Gastroenterologie, UnivesitI'astklinik Bochum

47. Firestein, Gary S. MD; and Zvaifler, Nathan J. MD : Anticytokine Therapy in Rheumatoid Arthritis, *The New England Journal of Medicine,* Volume 337, Number 3, July 17, 1997

48. Davies NM, Anderson KE :Clinical pharmacokinetics of diclofenac. Therapeutic insights and pitfalls. , 1997 Sep;33(3):184-213

49. Bondeson J: The mechanisms of action of disease-modifying antirheumatic drugs: a review with emphasis on macrophage signal transduction and the induction of proinflammatory cytokines, *Gen Pharmacol ,* 1997 Aug;29(2):127-150 1997 Aug;29(2):127-150

50. Biasi D, Caramaschi P, Carletto A, Pacor ML, Bambara LM: Safety of combination therapy with hydroxychloroquine, gold sodium thiomalate and Methotrexate in early rheumatoid arthritis. *Rev Rhum Engl Ed* 1997 Jul;64(7-9):521-522

51. Paul C, Le Tourneau A, Cayuela JM, Devidas A, Robert C, Molinie V, Dubertret L : Epstein-Barr

virus-associated lymphoproliferative disease during Methotrexate therapy for psoriasis. *Arch Dermatol* 1997 Jul;133(7):867-871

52. Phillips PE : Viral arthritis., *Curr Opin Rheumatol* 1997 Jul;9(4):337-344

53. Ferraccioli GF, Bambara LM, Ferraris M, Perpignano G, Cattaneo R, Porzio F, Accardo S, Mattara L, Zoppini A, Benucci M, Ostuni PA, Pasero G : Effects of cyclosporine on joint damage in rheumatoid arthritis. The Italian Rheumatologists Study Group on Rheumatoid Arthritis. *Clin Exp Rheumatol* 1997 May;15 Suppl 17:S83-S89

54. Conaghan PG, Lehmann T, Brooks P: Disease-modifying antirheumatic drugs. *Curr Opin Rheumatol* 1997 May;9(3):183-190

55. Schiff M: Emerging treatments for rheumatoid arthritis. *Am J Med* 1997 Jan 27;102(1A):11S-15S

56. Firestein GS, Nguyen K, Aupperle KR, Yeo M, Boyle DL, Zvaifler NJ: Apoptosis in rheumatoid arthritis: p53 overexpression in rheumatoid arthritis synovium. *Am J Pathol* 1996 Dec;149(6):2143-2151

57. Allan D. Kirk, David M. Harlan, Nicholas N. Armstrong, Thomas A. Davis, Yinchen Dong, Gary S. Gray, Xuening Hong, David Thomas, John H. Fechner Jr., and Stuart J. Knechtle : CTLA4-Ig and anti-CD40 ligand prevent renal allograft rejection in primates., *Proc. Natl. Acad. Sci.* USA Vol. 94, pp. 8789-8794, August 1997

58. Nilsson IM, Lee JC, Bremell T, Ryden C, Tarkowski A: The role of staphylococcal polysaccharide microcapsule expression in septicemia and septic arthritis. *Infect Immun* 1997 Oct;65(10):4216-4221

59. Burt RK : BMT for severe autoimmune diseases: an idea whose time has come. *Oncology (Huntingt)* 1997 Jul;11(7):1001-1014

60. Brooks PM : Hematopoietic stem cell transplantation for autoimmune diseases. , *Journal of Rheumatology, Suppl* 1997 May;48:19-22

61. Marmont AM : Stem cell transplantation for severe autoimmune disorders, with special reference to rheumatic diseases., *Journal of Rheumatology,* Suppl 1997 May;48:13-18

62. Hamilton JA, Biggs JC, Atkinson K, Brooks PM: Bone marrow transplantation in auto-immune disease., *Baillieres Clin Rheumatol* 1995 Nov;9(4):673-687

63. Snowden JA, Atkinson K, Kearney P, Brooks P, Biggs JC : Allogeneic bone marrow transplantation from a donor with severe active rheumatoid arthritis not resulting in adoptive transfer of disease to recipient., *Bone Marrow Transplant* 1997 Jul;20(1):71-73

64. Moreland LW, Baumgartner SW, Schiff MH, Tindall EA, Fleischmann RM, Weaver AL, Ettlinger RE, Cohen S, Koopman WJ, Mohler K, Widmer MB, Blosch CM : Treatment of rheumatoid arthritis with a recombinant human tumor necrosis factor receptor (p75)-Fc fusion protein., *N Engl J Med* 1997 Jul 17;337(3):141-147

65. Moreland LW, Margolies G, Heck LW Jr., Saway A, Blosch C, Hanna R, Koopman WJ: Recombinant soluble tumor necrosis factor receptor (p80) fusion protein: toxicity and dose finding trial in refractory rheumatoid arthritis. *Journal of Rheumatology* 1996 Nov;23(11):1849-1855

66. Moreland LW, Pratt PW, Mayes MD, Postlethwaite A, Weisman MH, Schnitzer T, Lightfoot R, Calabrese L, Zelinger DJ, Woody JN, et al : Double-blind, placebo-controlled multicenter trial using chimeric monoclonal anti-CD4 antibody, cM-T412, in rheumatoid arthritis patients receiving concomitant Methotrexate. *Arthritis Rheum* 1995 Nov;38(11):1581-1588

67. Adachi Y; Hinoda Y; Takahashi H; Nakagawa N; Sakamoto H; Itoh F; Endo T; Suzuki S; Imai K : Rheumatoid arthritis associated with ulcerative colitis., *J Gastroenterol*, 31(4):590-5 1996 Aug., First Department of Internal Medicine, Sapporo Medical University

68. Mosebach S; Tromm A; Wittenborg A; May B: Rheumatoid disorders in Crohn disease and ulcerative colitis. Dominance of non-inflammatory factors, *Leber Magen Darm*, 25(2):76, 79-85 1995 Mar

69. Toussirot E; Wendling D : Crohn's disease associated with seropositive rheumatoid arthritis., *Clin*

Exp Rheumatol, 15(3):307-11 1997 May-Jun

70. Breedveld FC : Early rheumatoid arthritis. Future treatment. *Baillieres Clin Rheumatol*, 11(1):83-96 1997 Feb

71. Haqqi TM; Qu XM; Anthony D; Ma J; Sy MS : Immunization with T cell receptor V beta chain peptides deletes pathogenic T cells and prevents the induction of collagen-induced arthritis in mice. *J Clin Invest*, 97(12):2849-58 1996 Jun 15

72. Kaandorp CJ; Van Schaardenburg D; Krijnen P; Habbema JD; van de Laar MA : Risk factors for septic arthritis in patients with joint disease. A prospective study. *Arthritis Rheum*, 38(12):1819-25 1995 Dec

73. Waisman A; Ruiz PJ; Hirschberg DL; Gelman A; Oksenberg JR; Brocke S; Mor F; Cohen IR; Steinman L : Suppressive vaccination with DNA encoding a variable region gene of the T-cell receptor prevents autoimmune encephalomyelitis and activates Th2 immunity, *Nat Med*, 2(8):899-905 1996 Aug

74. Li SG, Quayle AJ, Shen Y, Kjeldsen-Kragh J, Oftung F, Gupta RS, Natvig JB, Forre OT : Mycobacteria and human heat shock protein-specific Cytotoxic T lymphocytes in rheumatoid synovial inflammation. , *Arthritis Rheum* 1992 Mar;35(3):270-281

75. Trollmo C; Sollerman C; Carlsten H; Tarkowski A: The gut as an inductive site for synovial and extra-articular immune responses in rheumatoid arthritis , *Ann Rheum Dis*, 53(6):377-82 1994 Jun, Department of Clinical Immunology, University of G-oteborg, Sweden

76. Moreland LW, Heck LW Jr., Koopman WJ, Saway PA, Adamson TC, Fronek Z, O'Connor RD, Morgan EE, Diveley JP, Chieffo NM, et al : V beta 17 T-cell receptor peptide vaccine. Results of a phase I dose-finding study in patients with rheumatoid arthritis. *Ann N Y Acad Sci* 1995 Jul 7;756:211-214

77. Li SG, Quayle AJ, Shen Y, Kjeldsen-Kragh J, Oftung F, Gupta RS, Natvig JB, Forre OT: Mycobacteria and human heat shock protein-specific Cytotoxic T lymphocytes in rheumatoid synovial

inflammation. *Arthritis Rheum* 1992 Mar;35(3):270-281

78. Tanay A, Strober S, Logue GL, Schiffman G : Use of total lymphoid irradiation (TLI) in studies of the T cell-dependence of autoantibody production in rheumatoid arthritis., *J Immunol* 1984 Feb;132(2):1036-1040

79. Ogra PL, Herd JK : Arthritis associated with induced rubella infection. *J Immunol* 1971 Sep;107(3):810-813

80. Cobey MC : Rheumatoid allergic response to focal infection. Autogenous vaccine study for rheumatoid arthritis, *Clin Orthop* 1968 Jan;56:17-24

81. P. Tugwell, K. Bennett and M. Gent evaluated published evidence comparing Methotrexate with placebo. Guideline: American College of Physicians. Methotrexate in rheumatoid arthritis. *Ann Intern Med.* 1987;107:418-9.

82. Tugwell P, Bennett K, Gent M. : Methotrexate in rheumatoid arthritis: indications, contraindications, efficacy, and safety. *Ann Intern Med.* 1987;107:358-60.

83. Eric L Matteson: Recent clinical trials in the rheumatic diseases, *Current Opinion in Rheumatology* , Volume: 09, Issue: 02,Pages: 0095-0101

84. Cesar Ramos-Remus, Sami Bahlas, Orlando Vaca-Morales : Rheumatic features of gastrointestinal tract, hepatic, and pancreatic diseases, *Current Opinion in Rheumatology,* Volume: 09, Issue: 01, Pages: 0056-0061

85. Wolfe F: Comparative usefulness of C-reactive protein and erythrocyte sedimentation rate in patients with rheumatoid arthritis, *J Rheumatol* 1997 Aug;24(8):1477-85

86. Nikkari S; Puolakkainen M; Yli-Kerttula U; Luukkainen R; Lehtonen OP; Toivanen P: Ligase chain reaction in detection of Chlamydia DNA in synovial fluid cells. , *Br J Rheumatol* 1997 Jul;36(7):763-5

87. Jacobson JJ; Patel B; Asher G; Woolliscroft JO; Schaberg D : Oral staphylococcus in older subjects

with rheumatoid arthritis. *J Am Geriatr Soc* 1997 May;45(5):590-3

88. Coste J; Spira A; Clerc D; Paolaggi JB : Prediction of articular destruction in rheumatoid arthritis: disease activity markers revisited, *J Rheumatol* 1997 Jan;24(1):28-34

89. Conaghan PG; Brooks P: Disease-modifying antirheumatic drugs, including Methotrexate, gold, antimalarials, and D-Penicillamine. *Curr Opin Rheumatol* 1995 May;7(3):167-73

90. Agrawal S; Aggarwal A; Dabadghao S; Naik S; Misra R: Compound heterozygosity of HLA-DR4 and DR1 antigens in Asian Indians increases the risk of extra-articular features in rheumatoid arthritis. *Br J Rheumatol* 1995 Jan;34(1):41-4

91. Luqmani R; Sheeran T; Robinson M; Richardson K; Winkles J; Emery P: Systemic Cytokine measurements: their role in monitoring the response to therapy in patients with rheumatoid arthritis , *Clin Exp Rheumatol* 1994 Sep-Oct;12(5):503-8

92. Girgis L; Conaghan PG; Brooks P : Disease-modifying antirheumatic drugs, including Methotrexate, sulfasalazine, gold, antimalarials, and Penicillamine, *Curr Opin Rheumatol* 1994 May;6(3):252-61

93. Hayllar J; Smith T; Macpherson A; Price AB; Gumpel M; Bjarnason I : Nonsteroidal anti-inflammatory drug-induced small intestinal inflammation and blood loss. Effects of sulfasalazine and other disease-modifying antirheumatic drugs. , *Arthritis Rheum* 1994 Aug;37(8):1146-50

94. Ibe M; Rude B; Gerken G; Meyer zum Buschenfelde KH; Lohse AW: Coombs-negative severe hemolysis associated with hepatitis A. 1997 JZ *Gastroenterol*ul;35(7):567-9

95. Beutler AM; Schumacher HR Jr. : Reactive arthritis: is it a useful concept? *Br J Clin Pract* 1997 Apr-May;51(3):169-72

96. Buckley LM; Leib ES; Cartularo KS; Vacek PM; Cooper, SM : Effects of low dose Methotrexate on the bone mineral density of patients with rheumatoid arthritis. *J Rheumatol* 1997 Aug;24(8):1489-94, Medical College of Virginia, Virginia Commonwealth University.

97. Steinfeld S; Galle ; Struelens M; De Gheldre Y; Farber CM; Appelboom T; Van Vooren JP: Pyogenic arthritis caused by streptococcus equisimilis (group-C streptococcus) in a patient with AIDS, *Clin Rheumatol* 1997 May;16(3):314-6

98. Ferraccioli GF; Bambara LM; Ferraris M; Perpignano G; Cattaneo R; Porzio F; Accardo S; Mattara L; Zoppini A; Benucci M; Ostuni PA; Pasero G: Effects of cyclosporine on joint damage in rheumatoid arthritis, *Clin Exp Rheumatol* 1997 May-Jun;15 Suppl 17:S83-9

99. Toussirot E; Wendling D: Crohn's disease associated with seropositive rheumatoid arthritis. *Clin Exp Rheumatol* 1997 May-Jun;15(3):307-11

100. Ackermann B; Staege MS; Reske-Kunz AB; Dienes HP; Meyer:;zum Buschenfelde KH; Marker, Hermann E: Enterobacteria-infected T cells as antigen-presenting cells for Cytotoxic CD8 T cells: a contribution to the self-limitation of cellular immune reactions in reactive arthritis ? *J Infect Dis* 1997 May;175(5):1121-7

101. Cronstein BN: Molecular therapeutics. Methotrexate and its mechanism, *Arthritis Rheum* 1996 Dec;39(12):1951-60

102. Stein CM; Brooks RH; Pincus T: Effect of combination therapy with cyclosporine and Methotrexate on liver function test results in rheumatoid arthritis. *Arthritis Rheum* 1997 Sep;40(9):1721-3

103. Sandelin J; Harilainen A; Crone H; Hamberg P; Forssk;ahl B; Tamelander G : Local NSAID gel (eltenac) in the treatment of osteoarthritis of the knee. A double blind study comparing eltenac with oral diclofenac and placebo gel. *Scand J Rheumatol* 1997;26(4):287-92

104. Thalhammer F; Hollenstein U; Janata K; Knapp S; Koller R; Locker GJ; Staudinger T; Sunder-Plassmann G; Frass M; Burgmann H: A coincidence of disastrous accidents: Crohn's disease, agranulocytosis, and Clostridium septicum infection, *J Trauma* 1997 Sep;43(3):556-7

105. Zachariae H; Sogaard H; Heickendorff L: Methotrexate-induced liver cirrhosis. Clinical, histological and serological studies--a further10-year follow-up. *Dermatology* 1996;192(4):343-6

106. Bondeson J: The mechanisms of action of disease-modifying antirheumatic drugs: a review with emphasis on macrophage signal transduction and the induction of proinflammatory cytokines. *Gen Pharmacol* 1997 A;29(2):127-50

107. Richardson CE; Emery P: Innovative treatment approaches for rheumatoid arthritis. New cyclo-oxygenase and cytokine inhibitors. Innovative treatment approaches for rheumatoidarthritis. New cyclo-oxygenase and cytokine inhibitors. *Baillieres Clin Rheumatol* 1995 Nov;9(4):731-58

Appendix A

Searching for Information

There are many ways to obtain information on topics. One of course is the traditional library with its large collection of texts . This still a profitable method of obtaining information with some attention to detail and some work. If the information desired is Medical, then a medical school has the best texts, but they are very difficult to understand for the average layperson. Usually computers are provided to aid your search. There is an enormous amount of information and the staff will help. There is one sad fact: usually you cannot check out the material unless you have some affiliation with the Medical School such as doctor, nurse, student or , faculty. You can find some tiles of interest and take notes; if the book is very good, it may be in the Public Library run by your locality. Usually, this is not the case. Thus you must purchase the text if you want or refer to it for any great length of time.

Three are many large commercial bookstores that have excellent Medical reference sections and have books at very reasonable prices. The paperbacks are usually the lowest cost. If the topic is Arthritis, there are many good texts. Be wary of any text that has the words "Miracle Cure" and the like. If the book is from some University or Medical Center, it is usually worth the purchase. If the book is a hardcover edition, the price goes up, but not always. The medical reference texts cost more but contain more professional level information.

One of the very best sources of books is a Used Book Store near a large Medical University. The texts are not new, but the cost is usually very reasonable compared to new. If you have the funds, the Medical School bookstore is a very prolific source of information. The cost of the texts is quite high .

The Internet offers a very viable alternate and complimentary source of information on a vast array of topics. You will need some equipment for this but the cost is moderate. A computer with a modem is needed . The computer should have 16 MB of RAM (32 is recommended) , a cache memory, and a hard disk with about 500 MB capability or greater. The processor can be from 100 MHz to as much as 300 MHz; the lower end is usually adequate. The modem should be in the 33 Kbytes/sec. range, but higher is better if possible. A modern operating system is recommended. As an alternate approach, if you may

A Short Guide to Some Medical Sites on the Web

Most of these sites have copious information about **RA** and similar disorders. These are listed in no particular order. After you find something you like, use the links provided at the site to further the search. The locations are listed as http://www.*name*. This means HyperText Protocol Transfer (of Information which is almost always displayed as ordinary text and graphic images) . If you want to design a Web site HTTP is simply the display language used by the server (computer) . Use the open location command (click it with the mouse) and your Web server will find and connect to the location. Here is the list:

1. http://hopkins.med.jhu.edu Note: The www is **not** always used
2. http://text.arthritis.ca/news/
3. http://www.pslgroup.com/ARTHRITIS.HTM#Disease Note: Type these **exactly** as written
4. http://text.arthritis.ca/research/
5. http://hopkins.med.jhu.edu/NewsMedia/news.release.html
6. http://www.centerwatch.com/studies/LISTING.HTM
7. http://www.centerwatch.com/studies/CAT132.HTM
8. http://www.rxlist.com/
9. http://www.cc.nih.gov/
10. http://www@infonet.welch.jhu.edu/
11. http://www.cellpro.com/codesc.htm
12. http://www.cellpro.com/news.htm
13. http://www.netshop.net/%Ensardy/dancer/asmp.html
14. http://pharminfo.com/upcoming.html#mw
15. http://www.medmatrix.org/Spages/Rheumatology.asp
16. http://131.158.70.70/transplant.html
17. http://www.healthnet.ivi.com/hnews/bites/htm/9708nb.htm
18. http://igm.nlm.nih.gov/
19. http://www.duq.edu/PT/RA/TablefContents.htm
20. http://www.medconnect.com/cgi-bin/searchsites/pri?keywords=rheum.htm **Note: often these sites change name or are not available. The trick here is just to use the primary label which is for this site** http://www.medconnect.com. The name is medconnect; the .com means commercial. Other clues

are .gov=-government. Guess what .edu means ? Ans.: An educational site. OK how about .org (organization). Bet you didn't figure .ca . It means Canada not California.

21. http://www.arthritis.org/whats_new.shtml
22. http://easyweb.easynet.co.uk/~pgardiner/gmhotlist.htm
23. http://somi.ab.umd.edu/Microbiology/med_link.html

Another way to find sites is to use the Search devices with your Web browser such as Lycos, Yahoo,etc. Use a keyword for the search and if possible use two or more phrases to lower the hits. Allocate about 2 hours for this approach. This is one certain way of finding new stuff or sites ,but be prepared for massive listings. Learn to refine by using very specific terms. Use multiple entries. Just have Fun-that is part of the experience. All of the government sites have good information such as the National Institute of Health, MEDLINE,etc.. Skydancer in Canada is one of the best for Arthritis information. Any site that has a miracle cure-**Ignore.** The best time to search is off peak hours for the site. You will learn much simply by doing.

Appendix B

Special Care for the RA Patient

The special needs and care for the person with **RA** follow simple logic and well defined medical practice and techniques. Many books and pamphlets can help with this but this section will give some special techniques that I learned and was taught. The first consideration is your skin. This may sound silly to you but the skin is one of yours body's first lines of defense.

Skin Protection and Care-Things to Do

The many medication that are given to control the **RA** depress the Immune System and in addition many such as the Corticosteroids such as Prednisone, etc. and others cause the skin to be susceptible to damage from simple impacts such as bumping into stuff. You must make and wear the following. Make a cover for your lower arms and lower legs. This can be made of very thin leather and secured by Velcro. Thus any bumps or hits will have the impact absorbed by the leather instead of your skin. If you have had severe **RA** for more than 7 -9 years, this is **ultra important.** If you break the skin and at the same time cause a massive bruise, the site will become a focal area for invasion by microbes (various bacteria). The wound may appear to heal but this is not the case. It may appear to form a protective layer at first but later if you notice any puffiness or redness in the area of the wound or close to it, then a severe infection is developing. The weakened vascular structure plus the effects of the suppression of the Immune System by the medications will quickly produce a severely infected site-**See a doctor immediately !** If you wear the protection as instructed, this will be prevented. In an emergency, use an ACE bandage for protection.

If you do have an infected wound, see a doctor and follow directions. They will clean the wound and give you very specific instructions for the care of the wound. Use a 50% mixture of sterile water and 3 %hydrogen peroxide for cleaning. Do not rub. Use <u>sterile</u> gloves. Next clean with "Wound Cleaner "from a Medical Supply; this stuff is very good but cost about $17 but it works. Next, apply thin " sterile HydroGel". This is also available at a Medical supply depot. Now cover the wound site with sterile gauze all around the arm or leg. Do not tape directly to the skin. Use special Millipore plastic tape and tape the gauze to itself. Take the antibiotics as directed by the doctor. Gradually, you will see skin cells develop at the wound site. Do the wound dressing in the morning, late afternoon, and before bed. It will heal if you do as given herein. Next time wear the thin leather on your lower arms and lower legs (especially to protect the shin area.

In your home, sand and tape the edges of all the furniture. The edges can and will do damage. Keep a light on at night to see the hazards. Never walk in the dark. This may sound silly and like overkill but it works and will save you a lot of trouble. This only applies to patients with advanced severe RA.

Moving Around in Your House

There are many books and such that advise the patient on what is called daily living aids and procedures and devices that will help. Much of this can be obtained from the Arthritis Foundation at no cost- some is very inexpensive. Install devices to help you get out of bed and get up. Simple rubber straps attached to doors and structural points help. Use you arms and legs to raise yourself. If you have a two story house, you may have trouble climbing the stairs. Take your time and rest at intervals. You can bump your way down. They make lifts but they are very expensive at $5,000 **or more**, but they do work and make the task of getting up and down much easier. These stair lifts can be purchase used for much less at about $1000-1500 or so. It will take about 3 days to install. Another option is to move the bedroom to the lowest floor. If possible, a single story dwelling is preferred. The books will offer many tips such as chairs for the shower and additions to the tub.

Exercise

It is **vital** for your heart that you get some exercise each and every day. Walking is good as well as many other exercises described by the Arthritis Foundation. Next to walking immersion in a shallow pool is very good and swimming is even better. The YMCA or the YWCA have good pools for a minimum of cost. Health clubs are good but the cost is usually high. One option is the installation of a pool if you have the funds. The water must be kept warm at about 88-93 F . Avoid cold water and deep water unless you are a good swimmer; in any case, the water must be warm. An in place bicycle is good and can be purchase used for about $100 or less. Your lungs as well as your heart will greatly benefit from exercise. Of all that you or don't do, exercise is critical for a healthy heart and lungs.

Exercise may be difficult ; exercise may be painful. However, this daily activity is very important. No matter what, you must keep moving. If you allow yourself to sit or lie all day, much will occur that will be damaging. The body was not meant to be motionless and devoid of activity. Your heart and blood vessels not just your muscles **must** be exercised daily.

Appendix C

USC Public Law 105-115 (11/21/97)

Title I : Improving Regulation of Drugs

Title II : Improving Regulation of Devices

Title III: Improving Regulation Of Food

Food and Drug Modernization Act of 1997

* Title I: Improving Regulation of Drugs

* Title II: Improving Regulation of Devices

* Title III: Improving Regulation of Food

Food and Drug Administration Regulatory Modernization Act of 1997 - Title I: Improving Regulation of Drugs - Amends Federal Food, Drug, and Cosmetic Act (FDCA) provisions regarding fees relating to drugs to revise and add various definitions.

Makes the fee (currently, 50 percent of the fee) for human drug applications or supplements due on submission. Mandates a refund of 75 (currently, 50) percent if the application or supplement is refused for filing. Exempts from the fee: (1) an application for a drug for a rare condition (orphan drug) or a supplement proposing a new indication for a rare condition; and (2) supplements for indications for use in pediatric populations. Allows fee refund if an application or supplement is withdrawn. Modifies requirements regarding: (1) the annual prescription drug establishment fee; (2) the prescription drug product fee; (3) fee amounts; (4) fee adjustments; (5) fee waiver or reduction; (6) assessment of fees; and (7) crediting and availability of fees (including authorizing appropriations).

Terminates, on specified dates, the effectiveness of the amendments made by this paragraph.

(Sec. 102) Allows for additional deferred effective dates for the approval of certain new drug applications to allow for additional pediatric information developed by further studies. Mandates development, prioritization, publication, and annual updating of a list of approved drugs for which additional pediatric information may produce health benefits in the pediatric population. Prohibits granting a period of market exclusivity under these provisions after a specified date.

(Sec. 103) Directs the Secretary to facilitate development and expedite review of new drugs intended for serious conditions and demonstrating the potential to address unmet medical needs for those conditions. Terms such products "fast track products." Sets forth designation requirements and procedures.

(Sec. 104) Authorizes the Secretary of Health and Human Services to authorize the shipment of Investigational drugs for the diagnosis or treatment of a serious disease or condition in emergency situations.

Authorizes any person, through a licensed physician, to request, and any manufacturer or distributor to provide to the physician, such a drug if specified requirements are met.

Directs the Secretary, after submission of a protocol intended to provide

widespread access, to permit expanded access under a treatment Investigational new drug (IND) application if certain requirements are met.

(Sec. 105) Amends the Public Health Service Act to mandate a program in the National Institutes of Health (NIH) regarding information on research relating to the treatment, detection, and prevention of serious conditions, including establishing, and disseminating information from, a data bank of information on clinical trials for related drugs and biologicals. Authorizes appropriations.

(Sec. 106) Amends the FDCA to allow a manufacturer, in certain circumstances, to disseminate to health care practitioners, pharmacy benefit managers, health insurance insurers, group health plans, or government agencies certain information on the safety, effectiveness, or benefit of a use not described in the approved labeling of a drug if the manufacturer meets certain requirements. Allows the Secretary, on ordering a manufacturer to cease dissemination, to order the manufacturer to correct information that has been disseminated. Makes failure to comply

with this section a prohibited act. Terminates the effectiveness of the amendments made by this section on a specified date.

(Sec. 107) Mandates a study and report to specified congressional committees by the Comptroller General regarding the impact of, and the scientific issues raised by, section 106.

(Sec. 108) Mandates: (1) performance standards for the prompt review of supplemental applications for approved drugs; (2) final guidance's regarding the approval of such supplemental applications; (3) designation of an individual in each FDA center to encourage prompt review and work with sponsors to facilitate the development and submission of data to support such applications; and (4) programs and policies to foster collaboration between the FDA, the NIH, professional medical and scientific societies, and other persons regarding such applications.

(Sec. 109) Prohibits considering health care economic information provided to a formulary committee or similar entity false or misleading if the information directly relates to an indication approved under specified provisions of the Public Health Service Act (PHSA) for that drug and is based on competent and reliable scientific evidence. Declares that the requirements of specified PHSA provisions do not apply to information provided under this paragraph.

(Sec. 110) Declares that, if the Secretary determines that data from one clinical investigation and confirmatory evidence (obtained before or after the investigation) are sufficient to establish effectiveness, the Secretary may consider that data and evidence to constitute substantial evidence.

Amends the PHSA to mandate development of guidance on the inclusion of women and minorities in clinical trials.

(Sec. 111) Amends the FDCA to regulate new drug manufacturing changes, including requiring manufacturer validation of the effects of the change and setting forth separate requirements for major and non- major changes.

(Sec. 112) Allows a new drug clinical investigation to begin 30 days after specified materials have been submitted to the Secretary unless the Secretary prohibits conducting the investigation.

(Sec. 113) Mandates guidance that describes when abbreviated study reports may be submitted in lieu of full reports with a new drug application and with a biologics license application.

(Sec. 114) Modifies new drug requirements regarding: (1) application contents and review; and (2) the use of scientific advisory panels.

(Sec. 116) Directs the Secretary, if there is a scientific controversy between the Secretary and a sponsor, applicant, or manufacturer and no specific FDCA provision or regulation provides a right of review, to establish by regulation a procedure under which that party may request a review of the controversy by a scientific advisory panel.

(Sec. 117) Regulates the development, availability, and effect of guidance documents.

(Sec. 118) Declares a compounded positron emission tomography drug adulterated if it does not conform to the compounding standards and the official monographs of the United States Pharmacopoeia (but sets expiration dates for this provision). Mandates procedures for the approval of, and good manufacturing practice requirements regarding such drugs. Exempts, until specified dates, such drugs (if not adulterated) from new drug and abbreviated new drug approval requirements. Mandates termination of specified related notices and a related rule.

(Sec. 119) Mandates regulations regarding the approval of radiopharmaceuticals designed for diagnosis and monitoring of diseases and conditions.

(Sec. 120) Amends the Public Health Service Act (PHSA) to revise requirements regarding: (1) introducing biological products into interstate commerce, including related license approval and labeling requirements; and (2) inspection of biological product facilities. Modifies requirements regarding the certification of clinical laboratories.

(Sec. 121) Amends the FDCA to allow a pilot or other small facility to be used to demonstrate drug or animal drug safety and effectiveness.

(Sec. 122) Repeals provisions relating to the certification of drugs containing insulin or antibiotics. Allows insulin and antibiotic exports without regard to certain requirements. Declares that the antibiotic provision repeal does not apply to drugs that contain antibiotic drug ingredients that had approved or pending applications before enactment of this Act.

(Sec. 123) Sets forth an FDA mission statement. Mandates an annual report to specified congressional committees regarding FDA performance, staffing, and resources and listing bilateral and multinational meetings held by the FDA to reduce regulatory burdens, harmonize regulation, and seek reciprocal arrangements.

(Sec. 124) Mandates an information system to track applications and submissions to the FDA.

(Sec. 125) Mandates training for FDA employees on FDCA regulations and policies.

(Sec. 126) Mandates a demonstration program of grants for centers to conduct research regarding specified aspects of drugs. Authorizes appropriations.

(Sec. 127) Directs the Secretary to meet with representatives of other countries to discuss regulatory requirement harmonization.

(Sec. 128) Requires that an environmental impact statement prepared under specified regulations be considered to meet the requirements for a detailed statement under specified provisions of the National Environmental Policy Act of 1969.

(Sec. 129) Prohibits State and political subdivision requirements (inconsistent with this Act): (1) regarding the regulation of a nonprescription human drug or a cosmetic; and (2) not identical to a requirement of the FDCA, the Poison Prevention Packaging Act of 1970, or the Fair Packaging and Labeling Act, subject to exemptions and exclusions.

Adds references to nonprescription drugs to provisions authorizing inspections of places where drugs are manufactured, processed, packed, or held.

Modifies labeling requirements regarding the designation of drugs or devices by established names.

(Sec. 130) Mandates studies of: (1) mercury compounds intentionally introduced into drugs and foods; and (2) the effect on humans of mercury compounds in nasal sprays.

Mandates a study of the effect on humans of the use of elemental organic or inorganic mercury when offered for sale as a drug or dietary supplement. Directs the Secretary, if in the opinion of the Secretary such sale poses a threat to human health, to promulgate regulations restricting such sale. Prohibits such regulations, to the extent feasible, from unnecessarily interfering with the availability of mercury for use in religious ceremonies.

(Sec. 131) Requires a manufacturer that is the sole manufacturer of a drug, biological product, or device that is life supporting or sustaining or intended for the prevention of a debilitating disease or condition and that has been approved under specified provisions to notify the Secretary of a discontinuance of manufacturing of the drug or device. Directs the Secretary to distribute discontinuation information to appropriate physician and patient organizations.

Title II: Improving Regulation of Devices - Revises or imposes requirements regarding: (1) Investigational device exemptions; (2) expanded access procedures permitting the use of a device for the diagnosis, monitoring, or treatment of conditions that are life- threatening or could be irreversibly debilitating; (3) premarket approval requirements (mandating a device review priority); (4) humanitarian device exceptions; (5) safety and effectiveness device standards (allowing recognition of self-certifiable standards); (6) effectiveness determinations (as used in classifying devices); (7) reliance on postmarket controls to expedite classification; (8) substantial equivalence; (9) labeling (as affecting premarket approval); (10) supplemental applications; (11) premarket notification; (12) initial classification; (13) classification panels; and (14) premarket approval application review.

(Sec. 210) Mandates accreditation of persons to review and initially classify devices.

(Sec. 211) Mandates publication of a list of types of class III devices that are not subject to regulation under specified provisions and for which the Secretary has determined that premarket approval is unnecessary, requiring each to be reclassified into class II or class I.

(Sec. 212) Modifies requirements regarding: (1) device tracking; (2) postmarket surveillance; and (3) good manufacturing practice regulations (including foreign harmonization) and inspections.

(Sec. 215) Modifies recordkeeping and reporting requirements applicable to distributors. Removes reporting requirements regarding annual report filing certifications. Removes references to distributors from provisions relating to removals and corrections. Exempts wholesale distributors who do not manufacture, repackage, process, or relabel a device from provisions requiring annual registration of producers of drugs or devices. Modifies device user facility reporting requirements. Requires, for such facilities that are hospitals or nursing homes, user reporting regulations limiting user reporting to a user subset that constitutes a representative profile of user reports.

(Sec. 217) Prohibits considering a computer software product a device solely because its primary use is related to the provision of health care.

(Sec. 218) Removes from the list of prohibited acts provisions prohibiting, on a drug's or device's labeling or advertising, any suggestion that approval of an application is in effect under, or that the drug or device complies with, specified FDCA provisions.

(Sec. 219) Modifies FDA annual report content requirements.

(Sec. 220) Requires that the information system for tracking applications and submissions to the FDA requesting agency action (mandated by section 124 of this Act) permit, with regard to devices, access by applicants.

(Sec. 221) Declares that it is the sense of the Congress that the availability of a safe, effective, noninvasive glucose meter would greatly enhance the health and well-being of all people with diabetes.

Title III: Improving Regulation of Food - Amends provisions relating to food nutrition levels and health-related claims to allow certain regulations to be effective on publication at the discretion of the Secretary of Health and Human Services.

(Sec. 302) Modifies requirements regarding petitions to issue a regulation on health-related claims.

(Sec. 303) Allows a health or nutrient content claim not authorized by the Secretary if: (1) a U.S. governmental scientific body with public health protection or research responsibility directly relating to human nutrition or the National Academy of Sciences has published an authoritative statement, currently in effect, about the relationship to which the health claim refers or that identifies the nutrient level to which the nutrient claim refers; (2) a person has notified the Secretary; (3) the claim and food are in compliance with certain requirements; and (4) the claim is stated in a way that it is an accurate representation of the authoritative statement and in a way that it enables the public to understand the information and its significance.

(Sec. 305) Requires, if a nutrient claim is made and the food contains a nutrient at a level that increases to persons in the general population the risk of a disease or health-related condition that is diet-related, that the label contain, close to the claim, a statement referring to the nutrition information elsewhere on the label.

(Sec. 307) Mandates a: (1) final determination on any pending petition that would permit red meat irradiation; and (2) report to specified congressional committees regarding the process followed in reviewing that petition.

(Sec. 308) Prohibits: (1) implementation of any requirement banning, as an unapproved food additive, lead and cadmium based paints in the lip and rim area of glass and ceramic ware before one year after the requirement is published; and (2) banning such paints on glass and ceramic ware meeting specified criteria.

(Sec. 309) Deems a food contact substance (a substance used as a component of materials used in manufacturing, packing, packaging, transporting, or holding food, but not intended to have any technical effect in the food) unsafe and the food adulterated unless: (1) there is (and the substance is in conformity with) a regulation prescribing the conditions under which the substance may be safely used; or (2) the manufacturer or supplier has notified the Secretary of the identity and intended use of the substance and the manufacturer's or supplier's determination that the substance is safe under a specified standard.

(Sec. 310) Revises oleomargarine sale and labeling requirements. Repeals provisions relating to: (1) a congressional declaration of policy regarding oleomargarine sales; and (2) noncontravention of State oleomargarine laws.

Appendix D

Summary of Medications

This is a short summary of the current medications and treatments grouped current ; near future ; and under development.

Current

The first subgroup of medicines are the **NSAIDs** . These include:
The major side effects of all of these is moderate GI damage and in some cases ulcers. Work closely with your primary care provider in this selection. This list is not inclusive. No comment simply implies no experience with this **NSAID**.

NSAIDs

1. Aspirin or Buffered Aspirin- If you get relief stop here (Many people cannot tolerate Aspirin)
2. Feldene (Piroxicam)- Works but severe side effects
3. Relafen (Nabumetone)-Works without much side effect
4. Voltaren (Diclofenac sodium)-Some GI problems
5. Lodine (Etodolac)-Very good
6. Naprosyn (Naxproxen)-Good
7. Orudis (Ketoprofen)
8. Tolectin (Tolmetin sodium)
9. Indocin (Indomethacin) - Good
10. Clinoril (Sulindac)

This list is quite long and the best advice is whatever works with few side effects. For those unable to take Aspirin, use Acetaminophen . For pain, the use of Ultram (Tramadol) and/or Darvon (Propoxyphene) is effective. Anna tolerated Ultram much better with no side effects. Darvon gives dizziness and/or drowsiness. Of all that you can do-avoid Feldene. The price your body pays for relief is very high. These medicines help and give real relief-they provide no long term effect and some can be very damaging.

Corticosteroids

These medications do provide real relief and help for the patient. The price for this relief is high-very high. The first is noticeable weight gain. The next are elevated blood sugar, mood changes, and other similar effects. The other side effects take some time to appear but are of concern. These include thin skin, muscle weakness, cataracts, and other side effects that are of real concern. One of the greatest side effects is immune suppression such that infection is readily developed. The medicine works and does really help but the use should be the least hat will do the job. Generally, this should be the decision of your physician. If used long term this medication can not be suddenly stopped-the effect of this is death. The watchword here is use with care-great care.

1. Orasone or Deltasone (**Prednisone**) This was Anna's favorite. The others are used for injections and local site relief, etc. For simplicity the list will not be inclusive.

One other major side effect is osteoporosis which is very serious since really bad bone loss and embrittlement may follow. Thus, it is extremely important for those over 40, especially females, to take adequate calcium as a carbonate and Vitamin D. Some cases may require Premarin (conjugated estrogen) and the like. Thus taking one drug leads to the necessity for another one all having side effects.

DMARDS

This category of medicines includes those sometimes called the second line as used in military parlance. It was thought years ago that these medicines did indeed modify the progression of the disease-hence the designation. This now known not to be the case.

Gold and Gold Salts

The best of these is in my opinion the one with the lowest incidence of side effects. Thus **Ridura** (or Auranofin) or oral gold is **preferred**. The side effects include minor GI problems and skin rash. The injectable gold such as gold sodium thiomalate can give pronounced relief if one can tolerate the side effects. These side effects range from minor mouth problems to all of the skin detaching from the inner surfaces of the mouth (Anna had this). Other reactions are soreness of the tongue, skin rash, oral ulcers, and bleeding of the gums. Of great concern is possible bone marrow suppression. Thus, the medicine appears to be just as bad as the disease.

Penicillamine and Plaquenil

These drugs are listed next since the usual course of therapy follows to their use. Penicillamine may give some relief for a short while if the patient as severe **RA .** Plaquenil is good for Malaria-don't waste your time for **RA. Time is valuable ; you have a certain amount-don't waste it.**

Sulfasalazine

This may work if you have mild **RA.** This may also help for Chron's disease.

Methotrexate   (*Golden Boy*)

This medication really works and can produce dramatic improvement. If used in low dosage and with certain other treatments, this will help. Unfortunately, sometimes the liver damage is so severe that the medication must be stopped. If used early in the disease and with the proper dosage and combined with other DM drugs and NSAIDs, the improvement is dramatic. Sometimes, the damage to the liver is such that this must be stopped in about 2 years, sometimes, the patient can take this for up to 10 or more years. It is my opinion that his drug be used early at a low dosage and in combination with others for severe RA.

Cytotoxic Drugs

1. Azathioprine-(Imuran) This drug is used to block the immune system to prevent tissue rejection. It will work in the most severe RA if the patient can tolerate the side effects
2. Cyclophosphamine (Cytoxan) This drug is effective and will help but has serious side effects. The adverse reactions are anemia, bone marrow suppression, pulmonary fibrosis, elevated liver enzyme levels, and thromocytopenia and leukopenia.
3. Cyclosporine by Sandoz and others. This is used for the prevention of organ rejection after surgery. It is also very effective in **RA** . Some of the side effects are headache, nausea, edema, nephrotoxitic reactions, hepatoxity, and pain.

Nonspecific Help

There some medications that will not only help you to sleep but improve your outlook. Elavil , or amitriptyline hydrochloride, will help with sleep at night and is an antidepressant. Flexeril is good for muscle spasms and back problems and non specific spinal nerve problems.

New Drugs and Treatments

Current research has yielded a number of drugs and treatments. These are explained in the text but will be briefly presented here.

1. Thoracic Duct Drainage
2. Apheresis
3. Total Lymphoid Irradiation
4. Replace the whole supply of about 13 pints with blood from a healthy donor (at major Medical Research Facility)

5. Bone marrow transplantation for autoimmune diseases. Cellpro Technique

6. Enbrel by Immunex (may be available now)

7. Bispan by Inflazyme (available in some countries but not US)

8. COX-2 Inhibitor

9. Tenidap by Pfizer (available in Canada)

10. SelCID (US trademark) by Celgene

11. HC gp-39 by Anergen Technology

12. CD4 monoclonal antibody

13. MDX-33 by Medarex

14. Vaccine, comprised of mononuclear white cells from pregnant women

15. White blood cells (WBC) from spouses or special individuals (can be done by your local provider)

16. Colloral by Auto Immune Inc.

17. Arthotec

18. BClx-gamma by Boston Life Sciences

19. CTLA4-Ig (a B-7 specific fusion protein) and Anti-CD40 ligand (CD40L-5C8), Naval Research Institute (In development)

20. Neu-Sensamide by OXIGENE

21. Oxi-104 by OXIGENE

22. Anzemet by Hoechst Marion Rouse

23. Zenapax ® is also known as daclizumab by Roche (may be available now)

24. Interlukein-1 receptor antagonist (lab only so far)

25. NF-kappaB by Weizman Institute (lab only so far)

26. Recombinant human tumor necrosis factor receptor Fc fusion protein. (lab only)

27. Chimeric monoclonal anti-CD4 antibody, cM-T412

28. Immunization with T cell receptor V beta chain peptides (lab only)

29. Suppressive vaccination with DNA encoding a variable region gene of the T-cell receptor

30. V beta 17 T-cell receptor peptide vaccine (lab and limited trials so far)

31. Anadrol with Methotrexate and Folic acid

32. TMTX with calcium leucovorin

33. **ISIS 2302 for CD**

34. Diazaquinomycins A and B and AM-8042

This is what was found in this search. I feel certain that this list is much too short and much more is in the lab and unannounced. I am beginning to understand will update this information on a regular basis.

Appendix E

Mobility for the Severely Disabled

The care and needed services for the disabled can be effectively done with proper equipment and dedication. Many illness result in the patient being compromised physically and needing special care. Much of this is well known by health care professionals but the caregiver must learn. Of course persons can be hired to provide these services but the cost over an extended period of time can be prohibitive . Thus this section will try to educate the reader in the basics. Many good texts on nursing cover much of this in detail and should be consulted. If you know a nurse, try to get some basic instruction. If the patient is in the hospital, volunteer to stay after visiting hours and let the nurse instruct you in care techniques. Some will volunteer to do this when the patient are sleeping. Talk with the doctors as much as possible and try to learn at every opportunity.

Transport inside and outside the Home of the Patient

Many texts give detailed specifics on the care of the ill and special nursing care. Few or none tell you how to move the patient within their domain and to outside destinations such as the doctor or hospital. This will help and provide some insight as to what is needed and how to use the assistance devices.

Medicare will pay for much of these expenses if you are 65 or older. Unfortunately, if your patient is younger, much of what is needed is not covered under ordinary insurance plans and is very expensive. The invalid patient will eventually require a wheelchair. This is usually covered by insurance carriers at about 60 to 80 percent of retail cost. Some require that you pay rental and about 80% of the rental is paid and the payments accrue toward the acquisition of the wheel chair. The total cost or cost as given by many medical supply outlets is about $750 to $900. If you have to pay 40%, your cost will be $300 to $360. If you consult any industrial supply catalog, you will find that a wheelchair can be purchased from them for as low as $200. If you peruse classified ads , the cost can be as low as $50. The lesson is that any piece of needed medical equipment if covered by insurance or Medicare is price at about 3 to 4 times its value; or an inflation factor of 400%. These suppliers do a very profitable business at the expense of the healthcare providers. For some reason, this does not concern the insurance carriers or Medicare. Industrial suppliers supply the trade which is required by law to provide handicapped access to commercial and retail business. The normal laws of commerce do not apply to health care. This is precisely why it is so expensive. It is **NOT** expensive because you are sick. This is often quoted and the impression conveyed is that it is somehow the fault of the ill that they are ill and the high cost is justified. This not true; the cost for medical supplies is at least 4 times their retail cost if the market were not buoyed by the insurance carriers and Medicare. The same item, if it can be found in the industrial market, will be reasonable in cost.

Other medical care items will be required and the cost may truly overwhelm you. This can be dealt with for some items but not for items that can only be obtained from medical supply outlets. Inside the house, the patient may need a walker and a hospital bed and a potty. The walker can be obtained for about $80 ; the cost is competitive since any sources carry this item. A used one will be about $20. The potty must be purchase new ; this is also price competitive at about $60-$80 since many sources carry this item. A hospital bed can be very expensive but may be rented with the insurance covering about 60-80% of the rental fee. A new bed for home use will cost about $1800 ; a hospital grade unit will be about $ 5000. A used bed can be obtained for about $ 500 to $1000. There are companies that specialize in purchasing used or new surplus hospital beds ; they will resale the bed for about $800. Some of these companies are listed. Thus the market here is flexible and some judicious searching can result in big savings.

An example of a very simple device that is available commercially is the so called patient lift. The cost of this is about $1600. It is a frame with wheel and a hydraulic lift with a web for the patient. Now go to any automotive supply store and look for an engine lift ; the units are exactly the same except the engine lift is painted and is sells for $240. All you have to buy is the web sling for the patient. The list of devices that may be purchased elsewhere is quite extensive and the caregiver is advised to perform simple comparisons and shop where possible.

One big ticket item is vehicle transport for the infirm. If you call a commercial ambulance or transport , the cost is about $400 per trip. This can be very expensive if not completely covered and if your insurance carrier says that this is medically unnecessary. If your patient is under 65 , this is usually the case. Thus, if the person under care needs long term care and transport, then a vehicle of your own is indicated. This can be expensive at about $35,000 plus the cost of the wheelchair lift at about $5,000. Thus you need a quick loan for $40 grand or maybe not. Consult the classified in such sources as trading posts, classifieds, magazines that feature trucks for sale, etc. Most of this is available in such stores as 7-Eleven and the like. You can usually find a conversion van used for much less. It is possible to find a decent vehicle for less than $15,000 and an acceptable unit for less than $10K. If less, you will probably have to be careful or plan to redo the engine-about $2000. After you get the conversion van, remove the seats from behind the front seats. **Do not even consider a mini van-Not large enough to maneuver the wheelchair.** Removing the seats will require turning the seats strongly about 90 degrees and lifting. Two people are best for this unless you are very strong. Now make sure the carpet is intact and the rear bench seat is functional. The next step is to purchase or build wheelchair ramps. This will cost about $300 from an industrial supplier or as much as $800 from a source other than industrial. These may also be found in the classifieds for about $300. An electric wheelchair lift used can be obtained for about $1500-$2500 if you are willing to do the installation. Now equip the rear behind the rear seat such that the wheelchair can be stored here. Equip the space near the patient with porta -potty, oxygen, if needed, water, etc. All that is needed for a trip such that time is not a factor in the trip. Lastly, practice loading a wheel chair with weights to simulate the patient. You now can transport your patient almost anywhere and do not need the commercial carriers. This will be very satisfying for both you and your patient. **Also-GET A HANDICAP PLATE OR WIND SHIELD STICKER OR CARD FROM YOUR DMV.** You are now independent and will give your patient access to the outside world. This is most important for not only trips to the doctor but other more adventuresome trips such as to dinner, etc.

If the house is two stories, you will need to move the patient to a downstairs location. A new bedroom can be relocated on the ground floor. If this is not possible you must provide a means to transport the patient from the second floor to the first. Chair lifts may be purchased for about $5000 plus about $800 for installation. Used lifts may be found for about $1500. The installation will require some serious work but can be done by most in about three days.

The provision of mobility will do wonders for the patient. A sense of accomplishment for the caregiver will also be your reward.

Appendix F
Angels

This may seem to be a topic that is not scientific and found only in religious texts. However, some real help can be obtained by considering the nature of Angels. There are many texts including the Bible that fully explain Angels and most are familiar with these explanations and some of the texts. The following is from my own limited experience and may help.

Early in the text, I related how an Angel had spoke to me. It was most unusual and can not be proven or disproved . I was sleeping and something called to me in a very, very loud commanding voice. The best analogy is that of a father calling a child in a manner that compels attention. I awoke and saw no one and assumed it was Anna. She was sleeping soundly. Somewhat later, the same voice spoke again and said, " She has suffered enough ." I have never forgotten this and never will. Recently, after reading many texts and becoming very uninformed by any, I thought back about one experience that I have had that was most unusual.

It was late March and very cold and very windy. The grayness of the sky blended with that of the sea and the bleakness of the day was almost such that you merely wanted to stay indoors. This was not to be a pleasant day.

This was 1973, and I had recently just sold my sailboat . The new owners had been working on the boat all winter and wanted to sail it home. The new owners were just out of the Navy and seemed to fairly competent sailors. However, they picked a bad to sail, in my opinion. The water temperature was still in the 50's and the wind was about 25-30 knots. I greatly feared for their safety. Something or someone in my mind told me I **must** go with them or they would surely die. They was no assurance that a similar fate awaited me. Nevertheless, the feeling was so strong, that I insisted that I go with them and help. The voyage was about 25 miles and about half way there we would be about 12 miles from shore. My main worry was that the water was so cold that if something happened ,and they were in the water, their body heat loss would be such that in about 40-50 minutes, they would certainly be dead. Of course ,if I went I faced the same hazard. The message that I got was so strong that I went with them.

The boat was about 26 feet at the water line and 10 feet wide with two hulls-a large catamaran with cabin and sleeping quarters, etc. It had an engine and two large bilge pumps. I had been sailing it for about three years with no problems. The wind seemed to get stronger and stronger as we got farther and farther from shore. We tacked into the wind and made fairly good progress. It seemed to get colder and colder. I had on three layers of clothes including a heavy coat and was still cold. The waves got very high, and whitecaps were forming on the wave tops from the strong wind. You could only see water in all directions-we were about halfway to their port. Then, it happened-one of the hulls separated from the main structure. The gap was so large that you could see the sea. Massive quantities of water was coming in through the gap each time the boat reached the bottom or through of that wave. With the engine running and both pumps going, we were sinking. Death was almost certain for all of us.

I had an intuitive idea. Suppose I ran the boat before the wind with a small sail area. The sea would trail; i.e., the waves would follow the wind with us and the wind and sea at our rear. Even though the boat was large, it may surf with the extreme wind, and partially lift out of the water. I had done this years ago with small catamarans, but never with a large boat. The wind was at least 30 knots -maybe more. We turned and exposed a small mainsail and all of the forward small sail . It worked ! The hulls came out of the water and the boated surfed . The water no longer came through the open gap. We sailed back to the original port and docked. This was still a perilous journey and hand bailing and pumping had to be used as well as the bilge pumps. The wind was so severe that my skin had severe windburn with massive welts. About three hours later, the dock was in sight. We made it to the marina. Just about 15 minutes after securing the boat to its original docking, the boat sank. The windburn was so severe, it took about a week to recover. It was a miracle that we had made it back alive.

What prompted me to go on this perilous voyage ? How did I know to take the action that saved our lives ? Was an Angel with us ? What kept talking to me insisting that I go with the new owners ? I now think I know-it was a Guardian Angel. Some may not agree but the feelings were the same as those I have had recently. This does not prove or disprove Angelic presence , but in my mind, an Angel is a very real presence .

I read an article about a meeting of some of the world's most prominent physicists including Albert Einstein . Some of the wives were aware of approaching dinnertime and wondered what the fellows were doing. Einstein replied " We are trying to understand the nature of God ! "

As I read about nature and observe the immense complexity and concurrent simplicity, I am deeply impressed that this is not all by chance. Something has done this and has a real interest in us and our fate.

Angels must be God's messengers and immediate caregivers. Some humans, even, are sometimes in this category. Do something for someone that greatly helps the other and observe your feelings-There can be no greater happiness. We are here to help one another and to learn . **This is what we must do ; it is our destiny.**

Glossary

This is a list of some terms that you may or may not be familiar with. The explanation for each is directed toward the medical non professional and is not intended as a definitive text.

Analgesic- Any drug or medicine that that acts primarily to relieve pain such as aspirin.
Antibody- A substance created to destroy antigens or foreign organisms or substances.
Antigen- Anything that the body considers to be a threat ; may living such as bacteria or a virus or nonliving such as dead cells or harmful chemicals. With RA, your body is confused about who is the enemy and attacks itself.
Arthritis- A disease causing inflammation of the joints. These are many forms almost all cause inflammation of the joints, ligaments, tendons, and muscles. The arteries may also be affected. In some cases the eyes are affected. In some other cases , the skin or eyes are affected. Thus the term is not descriptive and must be used with a specific. The form that affects the bones is osteoarthritis.
Adrenal glands-Endocrine glands located just above kidneys
Antibiotic-A substance that can kill or inhibit microbe growth
Antibody-A protein known as immunoglobin that reacts with an antigen
Antitoxin-An antibody produced against a toxin
Arthritis-Inflammation of a joint or joints
Autoimmune disease- The immune system attacks its own host and causes great havoc. For unknown reasons at present, the immune system mistakes parts of the body as threats and attempts to eliminate or destroy these parts. (The term used is ABI or Army of the Berserk Immune which may not be scientific but is descriptive).

Blood Count-A test of a blood sample that measures white blood cells, red blood cells, and platelets.
Bacteria-Living organism with a single cell and a nucleus
B-cell-A white cell or lymphocyte formed in the bone marrow ; this cell forms antibodies to kill or inhibit antigens
Blood vessels-This has many forms from very large and carrying blood from the heart to the lungs and brain and the rest of the body -known as arteries to very small known as capillaries which have walls thin enough for transport of gases and nutrition, etc. The return vessels are known as veins which carry the blood back to the central pump called the heart.
Bone-Living tissue that is primarily of calcium compounds formed into very strong three dimensional

structural components. Prolonged bed rest and osteoarthritis can degrade these structures.

Cartilage-A very impact resistant and resilient material found at the ends of bonds in all joints. The cartilage protects the ends of the bones.

Chromosomes-Individual structures in the cell nucleus composed of DNA which a long chain of protein that carry essential information about self. Sometimes this information is not transferred correctly or changes permanently (mutation).

Collagen- The main component of connective tissues and cartilage.

Corticosteriods - Drugs related to the hormone cortisol ; also produced naturally by the adrenal glands. Cortisone such as prednisone is very common. Others fall into the gluccorticoid family. Prednisone and the like is taken orally ; many others are injected locally. Prolonged use can create as many problems as are solved. These drugs **cannot** be removed from a patient after prolonged use.

CD- Cluster of Differentiation : Cell surface markers with well defined biochemical structures and purpose. These are given designations according to function, location, and purpose. Consult the CD guide from the NIH. The list is for lymphocytes and is an indication of cellular function and expression. These are groups of so called monoclonal antibodies. These groups have adhesive properties and/or cell interaction and/or signal transmission. In a grossly simplified way, this how the T cells communicate.

Crohn's Disease- An inflammation of the intestine which may be trivial or may be life threatening and very severe. Severe RA may be associated with this disease.

Cytotoxic Drug or medicine- A class of drugs that kills dividing cells. These are widely used for Cancer but certain ones are also used for Autoimmune disease such as Imuran, etc.

DMARDS-Strong drugs such as methotrexate (Golden Boy) that are used when the so called first line drugs fail. With severe RA, this step should be taken almost immediately.

DNA-Deoxyribonucleic acid-The long double helix of paired proteins that carry the genetic information about self and self functions.

Erosion-Used in RA to denote loss of bone or cartilage in a joint. Caused by components of the immune system attacking collagen .

Endothelial cells-Cells lining the blood vessels

Enzyme-A protein or similar substance that accelerates a reaction, in this book, a biochemical reaction.

Estrogen-A hormone of the ovaries (effects such as those from estradiol)

ESR-Test to measure the rate at which red blood cells fall. If inflammation is present, the cells fall more rapidly. This test may be an indication of RA, etc. Your doctor will refer you to a specialist known as a Rheumatologist at this point.

Gene-One of a series of organized structures along the line of a chromosome

Hormone-A chemical made by the endocrine glands

HLA-Human Leukocyte Antigens-Histocompatability antigen genetic markers that may be associated with a predisposition to RA : HLA-DR4 . Others may predispose to other immune disorders.

Immunosupressive Drugs - Very potent drugs that decrease immune response. The ones called cytotoxic kill dividing cells. Methotrexate is sometimes included but Imuran and the like are always in this category. Used for RA and other severe forms of arthritis .

Immune system-The system that the body sets up to defend against foreign invaders or substances. Extremely sophisticated but may be confused or we may not understand this system very well.

Inflammation- A reaction to injury or infection or caused by RA and similar disorders. If injury or infection, then redness and swelling are prominent. May not be apparent in RA.

Immunoglobins-Antibodies and associated proteins

Joint- The bone connection-allows movement of fingers, knee, hips, legs, knees, hands, etc.

Joint aspiration-Removal of joint fluid (synovial).

Joint capsule- A fibrous sac that encases joint contents such as the ends of bones and the cartilage, etc. may be called the synovial sac since this is the fluid in the sac.

Lyme disease- A joint disease caused by deer ticks that may lead to RA. One of the few forms of arthritis with a known bacterial cause (Borrelia burgdorferi). This is treatable and a vaccine is now available.

Lymph and the glands-Pale yellow fluid ;the gland where the fluid is filtered. When infection is present, these become enlarged and noticeable.

Ligaments- Thick and strong connective tissue that joins bones

Lymphocyte-A small cell sometimes called white but may a T-cell or a B or other.

Macrophage-A large cell of the immune system with much capability.

Mutation-Alteration of a gene

Nodule -In RA, an accumulation of inflammatory tissue. These are under the skin but very visible.
NSAIDS- Non Steroidal Anti-Inflammatory Drugs :Drugs that reduce inflammation as well as pain. Aspirin and many others are in this category. Some may cause damage to the stomach or GI tract.

Ossification- Transformation of tissues into bone-like material.
Osteoarthritis-What the public thinks arthritis is. This is degenerative and causes loss of cartilage and bone mass. Also, severe loss of calcium in the bone and decrease in structure: (Osteoporosis)

Phagocyte-A cell that can ingest foreign microbes and even foreign substances
Thymus-The organ that participates in the education of the T cells (T lymphocytes); these cells learn to differentiate self from non self. Those cells not behaving properly are killed or programmed for self death (atopsis-cellar suicide). The B lymphocytes mature in the bone marrow. As adolescence is passed, this organ gets smaller and smaller.
Reactive arthritis-Arthritis resulting from infection but curiously, no live organism are found in the joints
Receptor-A molecule on the surface of a cell that will react with antigens, drugs, etc.
Rheumatoid factor-A protein associated with RA
RNA-The messenger form of DNA
RF - Rheumatoid Factor : An antibody found in large amounts in the blood in patients with RA.
Sciatica-Pain in the leg (severe) resulting from pressure on a nerve root usually from a protruding disc that compresses the nerve near the spinal column
T cell- A lymphocyte , may be formed in the thymus , later in life in the bone marrow
Tendons-Strong bands of connective tissue

Ulcerative Colitis-An inflammation of the intestine of unknown cause ; severe RA patients may have this disorder late in the course of the RA

Vasculitis- Inflammation of the blood vessels that can cause severe tissue damage. May occur with RA or may occur by itself.

Index

Made in United States
North Haven, CT
16 November 2025

82481798R00087